DANCING WITH THE MOUNTAINS

Alzheimer's, Angels, and the Appalachian Trail: A Journey of Spirit

By Paul Travers

For permissions, serialization, condensation, adaptions, or for our catalog of other publications Department.

Library of Congress Cataloging-in-Publication Data

Travers, Paul - 1951 -
Dancing with the Mountains by Paul Travers

Inspired by his father's dream of hiking the Appalachian Trail, Paul Travers hits the trail and finds that miracle in the healing power of America's sacred mountains.

1. Spiritual 2. Angels 3. Alzheimer's 4. Metaphysical
I. Travers, Paul - 1951 - II. Alzheimer's III. Metaphysical IV. Title

Library of Congress Catalog Card Number: 2020948554
ISBN: 9781940265940

Cover Art and Layout: Victoria Cooper Art
Book set in: Baskerville URW & Orpheus Pro
Book Design: Summer Garr
Published by:

PO Box 754, Huntsville, AR 72740
800-935-0045; fax 479-738-2448
WWW.OZARKMT.COM

Printed in the United States of America

To Frances and Herman,

loving parents whose lives were inspirational,

whose love was indestructible.

Author's Note

This book is a work of nonfiction. My trail journals, hand-scribbled notes, recollections, and personal observations were used to portray the events as they happened along the Appalachian Trail. My intent was to write my AT story, not publish my trail journal. Only a handful of names have been changed for privacy reasons. Due to publishing constraints, some of the people I met on the trail were omitted. Rest assured, their exclusion does not diminish their contribution to the story of my hike. They were trail angels who touched my spirit with their unique brand of trail magic. They were points of lights that guided me from Springer Mountain to Mount Katahdin. I will cherish those memories forever.

Contents

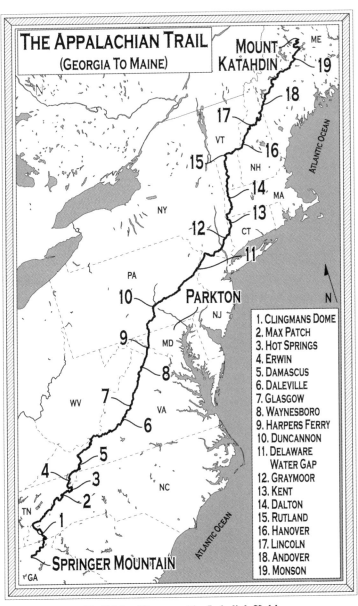

Trail Map Illustrated by Jedediah Kahl

Prologue
Daydream Believer

Whenever we go in the mountains, or indeed in any of God's wild fields, we find more than we seek. —John Muir

I came upon a child of God; he was walking along the road. And I asked him "Where are you going?" And this he told me. —Joni Mitchell from the song *"Woodstock"*

"One day we're going to hike the Appalachian Trail," my father boldly proclaimed on a summer afternoon in 1960. We were standing in the parking lot at Patapsco State Park, having returned from a brief hike along the Patapsco River. Those words struck me like a thunderbolt. My body tingled with excitement in the charged air. Invisible sparks flew from my fingertips. It didn't matter that I had never heard of the Appalachian Trail (AT). In my eight-year-old mind, it sounded like an exotic place with a mysterious Indian name that harkened back to the days of yore when mountain men roamed the great American wilderness.

For a Davy Crockett wannabe like myself, who religiously watched the eponymous television show, my father's proclamation was a career calling. All we had to do was go home and pack for the expedition. With a little luck, we could be on the trail by nightfall or surely by the crack of dawn. I didn't have a clue about who, what, where, how, or why of the AT. I knew it was only a matter of when, and when was simply a matter of time. With my whole life ahead of me, time was on my side, or so I thought.

Sadly, there was no hike that month, year, or decade. My father's interest in the trail could have been the result of a *National Geographic* article that he had read, or maybe it was a snippet of his own childhood dream that suddenly resurfaced for a few seconds. Twenty years later I returned to the state park as a park ranger and retraced those footsteps, but the Appalachian Trail was still no closer. Finally, nearly fifty years later, my dream was resurrected from the bottom of a desk drawer in my office.

While cleaning out my desk in anticipation of retiring, I came across a folder of news clippings that I had collected for nearly three decades. They were mostly articles about people that I knew in high school and college. Among the memories were a review of the new album by jazz vocalist Lisa Rich, the obituary of Tim "The Bulldog" Brannon, a high school teammate who rose to football fame at the University of Maryland, and a *Time* magazine report about the 1990 car bombing of Judy Bari, environmentalist, feminist, and Earth First organizer.

Finally, at the back of the folder, I plucked a tattered, yellowed newspaper article dating from 1984. To find out more about the AT, the columnist recommended the local library, local hiking clubs, and the Appalachian Trail Conservancy. I pondered the article for the next week before seeking the final seal of approval. Inspired by

Dennis Hopper's "living your dream" ads for Ameriprise Financial, I summoned the courage to approach my wife. In my mind, I was definitely not headed for bingo night and shuffleboard. I was out to prove that sixty was the new forty. I was going to fulfill the dream of a father and his son.

"I've got it," I brazenly proclaimed to Cathy, bursting through the front door of our home like a whirlwind.

"As long as it's not contagious, it's fine with me," she deadpanned.

"It's the fever, the white blaze fever. And it's not just for me; it's for us. We'll call it Herm's Hike (in honor of my father, Herman) and raise money for the Alzheimer's Association," I gushed, explaining my Appalachian Trail epiphany.

Over the recent months, we had talked seriously about my retirement. My father's battle with Alzheimer's had worn me to a frazzle. I couldn't see it, but friends and family members did, especially Cathy. Physically and emotionally, I was a walking zombie, mimicking the early signs of the disease. After three years as a caregiver, now was the time to simply drop everything and follow that dream. My family approved and I had no doubt my father would have driven me to Springer Mountain if he was able. Cathy had meticulously managed our finances to achieve a veneer of financial independence. The house, the cars, and the college educations for our daughters were paid. We were simple people with simple pleasures and passions. Who needed a retirement vacation to Hawaii or the Caribbean? Not me, and hopefully, not Cathy. We needed the road trip of a lifetime, namely 2,180 miles of mountain trail over fourteen states that would take six months to complete.

"Well, what about your foot?" Cathy inquired with a grimace.

My conversation stopped dead in its tracks. It wasn't a question about the foot. It was a question about the feet, specifically both of mine. In 2002, I had my left foot surgically repaired for "stiff toe." My nearly forty years of running, including the Boston Marathon, had taken its toll. The cartilage in the big toe joint had worn out, resulting in bone rubbing against bone. My smooth running stride had become a painful limp. Now six years later, I was limping with my left foot. I couldn't walk up the steps without pain. Hiking over the mountains for two thousand miles was impossible. My first step on the trail of my dream would be to the doctor's office.

"I'll call Dr. Joe the Toe and get it fixed," I replied confidently, trying to mask my true feelings. Joe the Toe was the moniker that I had affectionately given to my podiatrist. Although the first operation was successful, rehab was slow and painful. While contemplating a second operation, the mantra "No pain, no rain, no Maine" was already swirling in my head. I wondered if I would ever set foot on the trail.

Doc Joe was good on his word. Six months later after the operation, I was walking free of pain. My foot warranty was good for five million steps or more. As the bones gradually knitted, it felt as if I was walking on a bed of pebbles, but that sensation gradually dissipated over time. With that first painful step behind me, it was time to move forward and find a good pair of hiking boots and a sponsor for the hike.

In September, Cathy and I, sporting our new, top-of-the-line hiking boots, started a training program that consisted of biweekly local hikes in state parks with intermittent hikes on the AT in Maryland. Also that month, we found a sponsor for Herm's Hike with the Greater Maryland Chapter of the Alzheimer's Association. We had boots and a sponsor. All we needed now was hiking gear.

A quick inventory of our camping gear disclosed that we had enough equipment to survive a weekend trip in the backyard. Anything else would be flirting with disaster. Without serious upgrades, we'd be climbing Everest in tennis shoes and t-shirts. I had a 6 x 6 Coleman tent, an aluminum frame backpack from the early '80s, a multipurpose camp knife from my Davey Crockett days, a Marine Corps whistle, a Gore-Tex rain suit from my running days, and a polyester sleeping bag that barely fit in the trunk of a compact car. Cathy's contributions consisted of more tents and sleeping bags from her days as a Girl Scout leader and five camp irons to grill sandwiches and s'mores. If the AT ever hosted a s'mores festival, we would be in great demand.

By Christmas, we were in decent hiking shape and had completed our gear list with a Christmas shopping spree. Over the holiday, we decided that our first day on the AT would be March 31, 2009. I viewed the upcoming year ending in nine as a propitious omen. I graduated from high school in 1969, married in 1979, and would be retiring in 2009. The number nine was magical, mystical, spiritual, and highlighted in every major religion. The biblical number symbolized harmony, inspiration, perfection, and accomplishment of the divine will. Plus there would nine choirs of angels to watch over me. Even the pope gave his indirect blessing, having declared June 2008 to June 2009 as the Year of Saint Paul to honor the 2,000 birthday of my namesake. To make things even better, two of my favorites, baseball and the Beatles, were inspired by the number. I just hoped nine was my lucky number.

On New Year's Day, Cathy and I hiked comfortably and confidently in the woods for eight miles with a full backpack. Despite the optimism that increased daily, I couldn't shake the nagging thought that the Grim Reaper was hot on my heels. The decision to retire was a no-brainer. I had witnessed a number of retirement-eligible colleagues who never saw a retirement check after deciding to stick around for another year or two. Heart attacks, strokes, and cancer were the main culprits. I swore that it would never happen to me. I was going to take the money and run, or in this case hike. But despite my desire to prove that "60 is the new 40," I knew in my heart that it was just a euphemism for "over the hill" or "running out of time." While I embraced the dream of recapturing my youth, I had no illusions about its longevity. I was simply hoping for six months.

When I first entertained the idea of hiking the AT, I optimistically envisioned myself as halfway to the peak of "Mount Geezer" before the inevitable downhill slide. With age in mind, nothing seemed more apropos than an old hiker hiking and an old mountain range. Even though the Appalachian Mountains, which once rivaled the Alps and the Rockies in stature, were worn to a geological nub, they still represented a daunting physical challenge, especially to the senior hiker. With elevation gains and losses of nearly 465,000 feet, hiking the AT would be the equivalent of hiking Mount Everest (the world's highest peak at 29,029 feet) sixteen times. I also knew that lurking in that unfathomable fact about altitude was an emotional mountain of attitude that couldn't be equated. The physical and emotional peaks of the hike would touch the heavens; its physical and emotional valleys would descend into hell.

In the beginning, the thought of the Appalachian Trail as a spiritual journey had not entered my mind. By the end of my first week on the trail, I intuitively realized that moving forward would be not only a physical but also a spiritual transformation. While "the footpath for those who seek fellowship in the wilderness" is never advertised as a pilgrimage route, it can be for the worthy and wandering pilgrim. For me, the trail became my American version of the Camino de Santiago, the historic and iconic pilgrimage route in Spain.

In the end, it wasn't only the miles, but also the mountains that transformed me. Since the dawn of man, mountains have been prominent in worship and world religions. They have been revered as holy sanctuaries between heaven and earth where God awaits. Priests, poets, prophets, madmen, and mystics have journeyed to their summits for fulfillment. Much to my entertainment and education, I met a number of them along the trail, as I became one of them. Like our predecessors, we thought that we were searching for answers to timeless questions about the meaning of life. In reality, we were seeking to connect with the source of our being, whatever it may be called. Regardless of the cryptic theology or cosmology involved, one thing was certain. With almost three hundred mountains spread over 2,178 miles, the odds were in my favor for that chance encounter with the Creator.

Following in the footsteps of countless saints and sinners, I hiked mile after mile, mountain after mountain. With each step, I opened my heart in the presence of God's magical creation that we call Planet Earth. As my soul emptied in fear and anguish, it was filled with a stillness and silence only found in the divinity of nature. The mountain path became my road to a profound spiritual experience. I discovered the Appalachian Mountains were truly holy sanctuaries where wounded souls were healed and the mysteries of life deciphered. Ultimately, nature revealed itself not as the handiwork of God but the hand of God that leads each of us on a unique spiritual journey.

So journey with me on an American pilgrimage! Don't worry about your religious background. It's only a path that leads you to the trailhead of a spiritual awakening. All you have to do is lace up your hiking boots of hope and shoulder your backpack of faith filled with compassion and charity. Don't forget your hiking poles, your swords of salvation. And, most importantly, forget the miles and count the smiles!

Chapter 1

Spring Forth

(Parkton, MD, to Springer Mountain, GA)

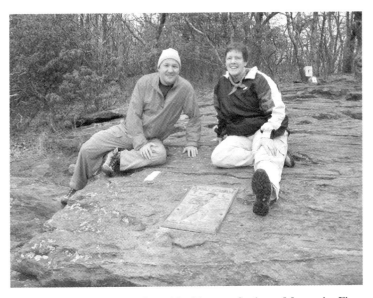

With Cathy (Brite) at the first white blaze on Springer Mountain. Five million steps to go!

Leaving my house on Sunday, March 30, 2009, I found my connection to singer Ray Charles. For over a year, I had Georgia on my mind, specifically Springer Mountain, the official start of the Appalachian Trail for north-bound hikers, commonly referred to as NOBOs. After locking the front door, Cathy and I walked hand-in-hand to the car. Herm's Hike, our Appalachian odyssey, had begun. Double checking the "don't forget" list, I opened the back of the SUV for a final inspection. Along with our hiking boots and hiking poles were two large plastic tubs containing camping food, hiking clothes, and miscellaneous hiking gear, such as batteries, bandannas, matches, toiletries, and first aid supplies.

Centered on the backseats, leaning toward the windows as if to catch a peek at the landscape, were two fully loaded backpacks with the latest in backpacking gear. The high-tech equipment came with a high price tag, but no expense was spared on a once-in-a-lifetime trip. Unlike my wife and I, our traveling partners looked completely at ease, their colors still bright and unblemished. At the end of the journey, I imagined they would be sullied, tattered, and frazzled like their hiking counterparts in the front seat.

As the engine purred to life, Cathy and I glanced at each other with raised eyebrows and tight smiles. "A kiss for luck and we're on our way," I sang softly, echoing the line of the Top 40 hit from the Carpenters in 1970, the quintessential wedding reception song of that era.

"We've only just begun," Cathy sang gleefully with a quick kiss on my cheek. In the early morning darkness, we rode in nervous silence, listening to a steady stream of "golden oldies" from the late '60s and early '70s, comfort music to ease the jitters.

"Well, what do you think?" I asked tentatively as we sped west on the interstate.

"We have to be crazy," Cathy replied smiling. "But it's a fun crazy," she added wryly. The truth had been spoken. If my wife had any doubts about the hike, she would have responded, "I don't think this is a good idea," or "Are you sure that you considered everything?"

Our enthusiasm spiked when we passed under the AT footbridge in Maryland. I honked the horn and waved at the sign above our heads that read "Appalachian Trail." In two and half months, I hoped to be waving to traffic as I crossed the bridge with a smile on my face, a song in my heart, and over a thousand miles on my boots. As the familiar miles heading west disappeared in the morning light, my thoughts rode shotgun down memory lane.

This was the road we had taken home as newlyweds, heading east from Colorado Springs in a compact sedan with a small U-Haul trailer that held our meager possessions. At the time, we had no jobs, no home, and no children. We only had each other. There were no mountains too high or rivers too wide that couldn't be conquered by love.

Today our love story had come full circle except now we were headed in the opposite direction with no jobs, no mortgage, and two adult daughters. Together we had scaled the mountains and swam the rivers that challenged everyday married life. As it was thirty years ago, the road was full of promise. Once again, we were alone in a car that was full of everything to start a new journey. I just hoped the mountains wouldn't be too high and the rivers too wide.

I don't remember the exact moment when the transformation began. All I knew was that it was happening, and it was happening inside the vehicle right next to me. Every time I glanced at Cathy, her countenance grew younger. I blinked wildly three or four times, and suddenly, the change was complete. Sitting next to me was a vivacious twenty-five-year-old brunette with sparkling blue eyes and a dazzling smile who claimed my heart when it was in the lost and found.

Cathy's words from earlier that morning echoed in my mind: "We have to be crazy, but it's a fun crazy." At that instant, I remembered those were her exact words as we headed to the justice of the peace in Colorado Springs during a blizzard on December 27, 1979. Ever the nervous groom, I spent the morning watching an endless stream of ominous storm clouds topple down from Pikes Peak and fill the town with snow.

Two days later as we headed back to Maryland, I watched the Rocky Mountains fade in the rearview mirror. With snow sparkling like diamonds littered across the landscape, I wondered if I would ever return to the mountains for another life-changing event. In 1979, the mountains had spoken and I had listened, even though I didn't fully understand the language. Now three decades later, the mountains were once again calling. And once again, I sensed magic in the air. Springer Mountain was pulling me like a magnet.

Heading southbound on I-64, my thoughts drifted back to my college days. As a young bohemian in the late '60s and early '70s, music and literature were the portals that transported me to southern Appalachia, a mystical place I considered the American Eden. Despite long hair and bell-bottomed jeans, I liked country music and its lonesome ballads with moaning steel guitars. So when country and bluegrass seeped into the folk pop scene, I was ecstatic. Following the lead of musicians like James Taylor, I replaced my tie-dye t-shirts and sandals with flannel plaids and work boots. The down-home, country trend suited my personality despite being a city slicker from Baltimore who had never tilled an acre behind a horse and a plow. Now that I had the right look, I needed to find the right books, a much more difficult task than new shirts and shoes.

As an English major, the English Romantics bored me to death. I wanted to study the American Romantics, those writers who harvested their words in the shadows of the Blue Ridge Mountains. On the bookshelf in my dorm room, I replaced Blake, Wordsworth, and Coleridge with Thomas Wolfe (*Look Homeward, Angel*), James Still (*River of Earth*), and later Anne Dillard (*Pilgrim at Tinker Creek*). My new literary friends spoke the language of the Appalachian mountain people; they spoke the tongue of my adopted tribe.

Hours later we turned east on I-40 and crossed the backbone of the Great Smoky Mountains, skirting the northern edge of the national park. At one of the overlooks, we pulled over to stretch our legs and savor our first view of the Smokies. Somewhere in the mountain vista were fourteen peaks with elevations above 6,000 feet. One after another, the green mountains rolled like a giant wave before disappearing into the dull white haze of the late afternoon. The portrait of this American wilderness was mesmerizing and frightening. Our tight smiles quickly turned to frowns when we realized the dull white haze was actually snow. Winter still gripped the peaks. We hustled back to the warmth of the car and hoped the "real" spring was around the corner.

Late in the afternoon, we arrived at Franklin, North Carolina, our jumping-off point for the hike. The

Sapphire Motel, home for the night, was eerily quiet and empty. Cathy and I spotted two women unloading backpacks from a car and three young men on the balcony with hiking boots and beers in hand. After scheduling our ride to Springer Mountain in the morning, I asked the clerk about the lack of hikers. "Just missed 'em. They went home or back to the trail this morning," he drawled with a southern twang before explaining the annual April Hiker Fool Bash, a weekend festival featuring food, music, outdoor exhibits, and, of course, hikers.

"Kind of sorry I missed it," I said casually, feigning disappointment. Cathy and I looked at each other and smiled with a nod. At least, we would have one good night's sleep before we hit the trail.

After dinner at a nearby Mexican restaurant, our last chance to load up on calories and carbohydrates, we returned to our room for a final check. After an hour of nervously unloading and loading our backpacks, we wearily climbed into bed with visions of the AT dancing in our heads.

At 7 o'clock the next morning, our driver was dutifully waiting for us at the motel office. Before leaving, we curiously checked the hiker's box in the lobby. The box, a communal bin where hikers unloaded trail items for fellow hikers, was relatively bare. No doubt, it was still too early in the season. In the age of ultralight hiking, the box had become a mini-dumpster filled with antiquities from novice hikers, such as metal canteens, frying pans, canned goods, kitchen cutlery, and cotton clothing. On the plus side, the box could be a treasure chest or convenience store. If a hiker was lucky, the bin could replace lost or forgotten items, such as gloves, socks, water bottles, ibuprofen, blister aids, and packets of freeze-dried food.

Cathy and I threw our backpacks into the back of the van and settled in for the ride. "How far to Springer?" I asked our driver excitedly.

"About 120 miles or so. Should take us a good three hours. Lots of logging roads in the mountains," Dave replied sleepily, nursing a cup of coffee.

Staring out the window in silence, I pondered the new math for hikers. On the trail, time and distance had new correlations. What took three hours to drive would take about two weeks to hike. The road mileage from Springer Mountain to Mount Katahdin, the northern terminus in Maine, was 1,423.4 miles, requiring twenty-three hours and thirty-six minutes. According to my 2009 AT companion book, the thru-hiker's bible, the trail mileage was 2,178.3, requiring approximately six months of hiking in my case. Distance would now be measured in miles per day, not miles per hour. Trail math required new variables, such as the hiker's age, weight of the backpack, trail elevation, number of blisters, equipment failure, dates of trail festivals, zero days, and weather events. Absolute values were how much money you needed for a night in town; radicals were your fellow hikers, and fractions were how much food you had before a resupply. Logarithms were downed trees that blocked your way. Sines and cosines were the next white blaze or trail marker. That was the only math that needed to be understood.

Heading south toward Neel Gap on US 129, we passed a historical marker for the boyhood home of Byron Herbert Reece. I caught a brief glimpse of the farm before we turned off the highway and entered a maze of logging roads. I had accidentally discovered the acclaimed Appalachian poet, novelist, and farmer while surfing the Internet for information about the trail. I was captivated by his genius. His haunting poems about life, love, and death in Appalachia were a prism for the melancholic beauty of nature that surrounded his life. I wished that I had met him earlier. His works would have found a prominent place in my dorm room bookcase.

As the van slowly gained altitude and plunged deeper into the dark woods, I spotted a group of camouflaged soldiers standing next to communication vehicles parked along the road. They were from nearby Camp Frank D. Merrill, heralded as the toughest combat school in the world. The "camp" was described as a place where small unit leaders develop leadership and survival skills in a tactically realistic mountain environment under mental and physical conditions found in combat. *That should be the prologue to my AT companion guide*, I thought. *Just substitute "Appalachian Trail" for "camp."*

"Looks like they're headed out for a search-and-rescue mission. Must be a lost NOBO (northbounder)," I joked as the soldiers disappeared into the forest.

"Let's hope not because we're only a few miles from Springer. But it would be one heck of a good story," Dave laughed. And then on cue, he proceeded to regale us with tales about hikers that he had returned. Some wannabe thru-hikers jumped out of the van, took a look around, and jumped right back inside. Others called for a ride home after one day on the trail. A few turned around before reaching the parking area at Springer Mountain.

Cathy and I chuckled at the stories, but they were not exactly the words of encouragement for his current load of nervous novices. Right then, I decided that no matter what happened today, we would spend at least one night on the mountain before calling Dave and heading home.

Minutes later, we stopped at a desolate, gravel parking lot. "This is it. Springer is about a mile that way," Dave said exiting the vehicle and pointing south to a path in the naked trees. "If you need any kind of help, you have Ron's (Haven) number. Have a safe hike. See you in Franklin."

Cathy and I grabbed our backpacks, ensuring that nothing was left behind, tipped Dave handsomely (his trail stories alone were worth the price of the ride), and said good-bye. As Dave climbed into the driver's seat, a woman and her teenage son emerged from the tree line and approached the van. Crossing the road, we heard the woman haggling for a cheaper rate. It was not forthcoming. There was no discount for quitters. They had spent one night on the mountain. Cathy and I stared in silence with furrowed brows as the van disappeared down the road. Dave had two new customers, one miffed mother and her relieved son, and another trail story. Wannabe hikers quickly learned that while the trail was free, anything outside the eighteen-inch-wide path had a price to pay in more ways than one.

With adrenalin pumping, Cathy and I stepped cautiously along the rocky trail that led to Springer Mountain. The last thing we wanted to do was become casualties before our first official step on the trail. I was sure that Dave had that story in his repertoire. About a half an hour later, we turned a corner and stepped onto a rocky outcropping. I recognized it immediately as

Springer Mountain. Cathy and I stopped to savor the view.

"Spring forth from Springer Mountain in the spring!" I exclaimed, tapping the rocks with my hiking pole. The first mountain on the trail was named for either William Springer, an early settler appointed by the governor in 1833 to implement legislation to aid the Indians, or John Springer, the first Presbyterian minister ordained in Georgia in 1790. For unknown reasons, the locals once called it Penitentiary Mountain, a name that seemed appropriate to many hikers, most likely those who returned with Dave.

We dropped our backpacks and scrambled down to the rocks where two bronze plaques with greenish tint announced the official start of the AT. Next to the first white blaze on the trail was a plaque from the Georgia Appalachian Trail Club, dated 1934. Depicting the silhouette of a hiker, it said, "A Footpath for Those who seek Fellowship with the Wilderness." Simply and elegantly stated, the mantra was a powerful gospel of nature that could change your life. The other plaque from the US Forest Service, dated 1993, displayed a map of the eastern states with the words: "Appalachian National Scenic Trail, Springer Mountain – Elevation 3762', Southern Terminus, Chattahoochee National Forest."

As we reached for our cameras to document our arrival, a voice from above startled us. Turning our heads, we spotted an older gentleman sitting in a folding chair. Roger Dunton, ridge runner, thru-hiker, and official AT greeter, cordially welcomed us to the mountain. With a gaunt face, a white beard, and white hair stuffed under a baseball cap, he was a dead-ringer for Gandalf from the movie *The Hobbit.*

"Folks like to register for your hike?" Roger asked in a friendly voice as he walked toward us with a ledger in his hand. He quickly recorded the date, our names, hometown, and trail names if any. The last request caught us by surprise. Cathy and I hurriedly discussed possible names, unaware that fellow hikers usually bestowed trail names. Cathy chose Rainbow Brite, the lead character in the animated television series. I picked Rain Man because I liked to walk, not necessarily hike in the rain, or so I thought I did. Cathy had a winner. What's not to like about someone who battles the forces of darkness to bring the color to the world, mainly the colors of hope and happiness. In the days to come, Rainbow Brite would be shortened to Brite. Rain Man would be a short-lived moniker due to the weather.

After a pep talk and short lecture about the "leave no trace" philosophy, Roger took our ceremonial pictures at the plaques. Engaging in small talk, he said that he lived ten days on the mountain with four days off. "How long have you been doing this?" I inquired curiously.

"Many sleeps," he answered quickly, flashing a sly grin. Cathy and I nodded our heads and laughed. We had just met our first trail legend, Many Sleeps, the gatekeeper of Springer Mountain.

After kissing the plaques and touching the first white blaze (the ubiquitous 2 x 6-inch white rectangle painted on trees, rocks, and posts that marked the trail), Cathy and I shouldered our backpacks. The day was growing short, and we still had an eight-mile hike to our first shelter. We retraced our steps with a sense of relief, not urgency. No matter what happened from this step forward, we were officially hiking the Appalachian Trail.

In the parking lot, we noticed a stranger loitering underneath the AT kiosk next to the trail. Dressed in green pants, green jacket, and a nondescript baseball cap, the thin, middle-aged man looked like an employee of the forest service. Staring straight ahead with his arms at his side, he casually glanced from side to side as if waiting for a bus. He was actually waiting for hikers. After exchanging greetings, Scott informed us that he was a former thru-hiker who lived nearby. Every year, if he wasn't hiking, he stopped along the trail to meet and greet the newest class. His trail name was Pilgrim. As we spoke, I wracked my brain trying to determine when and where I had heard that name.

"Where do you hail from?" Scott asked.

"Maryland, just north of Baltimore," I replied.

"Anywhere near Parkton?"

"Right in the heart of Parkton. Just about a mile and a half from hike and bike trail."

"Then you know Mike Wingeart or Wing-Heart?"

"Know him. He was my trail guru," I chuckled in amazement. "Now I remember the trail name. You're his hiking partner."

Wing-Heart was my first trail angel. At his house, I inspected his extensive inventory of hiking gear, asked the most novice questions, and borrowed books and DVDs from his AT library. Scott was amazed that I could visit Mike before sunset and leave before sunrise. The loquacious and gracious Wing-Heart was the proverbial walking AT encyclopedia.

As Cathy and I headed down the trail, I was remiss that I didn't ask Scott about the origin of his trail name. Was he related to the first settlers who arrived on the *Mayflower* or had he walked the El Camino de Santiago? No matter, the first person that Brite and I had met on the trail was a self-described pilgrim. I couldn't help but wonder if I was a pilgrim, a pupil, or a pretender. But there was no need to worry at the moment. I had six months to answer that question.

Chapter 2
Appalachian Tsunami
(Springer Mountain to Neel Gap, GA)

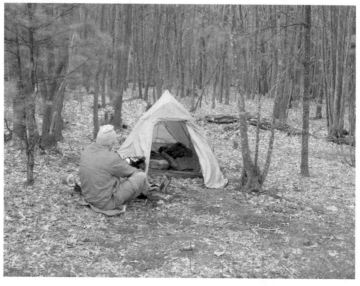

Auntie Agnes B&B, room for two, maybe, but waterproof.

Brite and I hiked at a leisurely pace through a rolling forest of pine and hemlock and tunnels of rhododendron thickets, the proverbial "green tunnel." About every two miles, we stopped to rest, throwing off the backpacks in ecstasy and grabbing mouthfuls of gorp, the ubiquitous trail snack of granola, nuts, dried fruit, and chocolate. The weather was cool and cloudy with the temperatures in the low 50s, a perfect hiking day.

That first day we averaged a little more than two miles an hour. By late afternoon, we reached our home for the evening in a light shower and falling temperatures. Hawk Mountain Shelter, your typical three-sided wooden slab structure with an upper berth, looked inviting, but there was no room at the inn. Instead of sleeping under a wooden roof, Brite and I settled for a night with Auntie Agnes, the name we lovingly gave to our Big Agnes tent.

After pitching our tent, we gathered around the communal picnic table to chat and dine with our fellow hikers. Names and trail names were eagerly exchanged and discussed, but the main topic was gear as it would be for the entire hike. Our first dinner on the trail was freeze-dried chicken chow mein followed by a chocolate chip Pop Tart for dessert. All of it washed down with powdered lemonade. Gourmet dining was never on any shelter menus.

By 8 o'clock, hikers were seeking refuge in their sleeping bags from the chilled mountain air. Brite and I retreated to our four walls of high-tech, lightweight, silicone-treated, rip-stop nylon with a waterproof polyurethane coating. It was advertised to sleep two, but it didn't say two of what—two trolls or two hobbits, maybe. In our case, the actual capacity was one and a half, but we were quick to adapt. In minutes, we mastered the art of changing from hiking to sleeping clothes inside a sleeping bag. Seconds later, we were toasty warm, nestled in beds of goose down. After critiquing our first day on the trail, we drifted off to a well-deserved sleep as faint voices from the shelter faded in the night. I felt it had been an auspicious start. I only hoped Brite thought the same.

Hours later my slumber was rudely interrupted by soft muffled pings, the unmistakable sound of rain against the tent. I grabbed my headlight and did a quick inspection. No drips or wet spots were evident. The morning brought more good news. The tent was still bone-dry. Auntie Agnes had passed the initial trial by water.

By dawn, the rain had stopped and the sounds of the morning campground filled the air. Camp stoves hissed under pots of boiling water for coffee and oatmeal while zippers raced along tents, jackets, and backpacks.

With our sleeping hoods drawn tightly around our heads, Brite and I rolled over to face each other and our inevitable fate. We had to break camp quickly and hit the trail early for a space at the next shelter. But on a cold mountain morning, there was nothing more enticing than a warm bed. Reluctantly, we clumsily changed into our hiking clothes and crawled out the front flap for morning roll call with our fellow hikers.

At 7:30 a.m., after a breakfast of coffee and Pop Tarts, Brite and I shouldered our backpacks and headed north. Chasing the next white blaze was now our morning commute, and the trail was our workplace. Our job was simply to hike as many miles as possible. Before clocking in and clocking out, we had the monotonous task of making and breaking camp. On the positive side, there were no alarm clocks, deadlines, meetings, phone calls, or obnoxious bosses. And you didn't have to worry about what clothes to wear. Every day was now a casual Friday.

On our second day, a morning shower created a cold dampness that seeped through every layer of clothing. From the valley below, a light wind floated a fog bank that limited our visibility. For our psyche, it was best that we didn't see what was ahead. The mountains were flexing their mighty muscles, and we were hiking over the bulging biceps. The gentle rolling ridges of the previous day had been compressed into nature's rollercoaster. All day long we rode the mountains to Gooch Mountain Shelter, gamely conquering the detested PUDs, pointless ups and downs that characterized the trail.

We covered only seven miles but were satisfied with our progress. However slow, it was steady. At the shelter, we claimed the last two spaces at the front. At the time, it didn't seem like the ideal location, but if either of us had to heed the call of nature during the night, we could easily grab a headlight and step outside.

Dinner that evening, another freeze-dried entrée, included entertainment, the AT version of a floorshow. Auditions were being held for homemade, portable alcohol stoves. One by one, the four contestants confidently approached the picnic table, now center stage, eager to prove themselves as survivalists and inventors. To the jeers and cheers of their fellow hikers, these fire-producing daredevils of dinner carefully assembled their metal contraptions with a running commentary about the engineering and environmental advantages of their stove over a commercial one. Wind funnels, wind barriers, wind flaps, fuel injection systems, and industrial-sized fuel canisters of highly combustible white alcohol that could launch a space shuttle were some of the technological features on display.

As the audience held their collective breath, the contestants one by one carefully ignited their devices. Flames leaped to the heavens with a beastly roar as fiery, orange waves rolled across the table. Contestants and hikers scrambled to rescue themselves, their gear, and their dinner. Cries of "Oohs" and "Aahs" and shouts of "Assholes" rang out with subdued clapping.

To the relief of everyone who feared the shelter would go up in flames, the fires quickly burned out. Luckily, all that remained was a scorched picnic table. The dinner lesson was not lost on some of the hikers, including me. Homemade was not always well made; windproof was not always foolproof; and penny wise was usually pound foolish on the trail. I smiled at Brite and pointed to my camp stove on the shelter floor. My pocket-sized, ultralight backpacking stove was "the little engine that could." It was the brunt of many jokes, but no one laughed when I fired it up. No fuss, no mess, and no assembly or fire extinguisher required. In the back of my mind, I wondered what would have happened if one of these camp stove magicians had accidently set themselves on fire. It was a question that I hoped was never answered.

Later that evening, Brite and I gathered around the picnic table for the nightly bull session. We quickly learned that hikers were natural-born storytellers who could spin a good yarn in a dorm room, barroom, or boardroom. Lost jobs, lost spouses, lost dreams, and just plain lost in today's world were the main reasons for hitting the trail. One of the more eloquent speakers was an affable young man in his mid-twenties with the self-proclaimed trail name of Rehab. He was hiking the trifecta, hoping to lose weight, quit smoking, and stop drinking before his impending wedding. A week later he disappeared from the trail, fate unknown. It was amazing to think that so many lost souls were hoping to hike over

2,000 miles in the wilderness to find resolution and absolution. But who was I to judge. I was now part of this lost tribe of dreamers and doers.

The only thing missing from a perfect trail night was a campfire. All winter, I had pictured myself basking in the warm glow of a roaring fire with Brite by my side. Unfortunately, this backpacking staple rarely materialized during the first month on the trail. The area around the shelter had been picked clean of every sliver of combustible wood. Scavenger parties returned with dry rot, water-soaked logs that wouldn't burn in hell. So instead of huddling around a campfire, we huddled around a picnic table, dressed in gloves, knit hats, and jackets and shaking our arms and legs to keep the blood flowing.

As the night passed, the conversation whimsically drifted toward Mount Katahdin, now only 2,160 miles to the north. Most were confident they would be summiting the final mountain in six months or less. I counted nineteen faces in the evening shadows and realized that only four or five would reach the northern terminus. That was the average. Just about anything could end a hike: death, disease, famine, broken bones, broken hearts, bear attack, snakebite, spider bite, weather, and just plain bad luck like running out of money or time. Seemingly, everyone knew someone who had endured these misfortunes, the AT's version of the plagues of Egypt. Fact was always stranger than fiction on the AT, a revelation that was waiting to be manifested.

By 9 o'clock, the last headlight had been extinguished, and Brite and I settled in for a good night's sleep. Minutes later, my eyes instantly popped wide open at the cacophony of wet snores, dry snores, sucking snores, gushing snores, and even a few death rattles! Wheezing, hacking, grinding, and sawing! I had no doubt that people in the valley could hear the racket.

I briefly panicked, but quickly remembered the fatherly advice of Wing-Heart. After a few seconds of fumbling in the darkness, I found my earplugs. Wing-Heart had warned me to steer clear of any hiker with the word "saw" in his name, such as Jigsaw, Buzz Saw, and Sawmill. That was the calling card for a professional snorer who sang the song of the lumberjack.

My hiking partner slept soundly as usual. I was convinced that nothing short of a volcanic eruption beneath the tent or a marching band parading through the campsite could disturb Brite's sleep. Oh, how I envied her. Nothing but imminent danger would be her wake-up call. Tempting fate, my theory about her would be tested shortly.

The following morning dawned cold, dreary, and wet. Our sleeping bags were damp from the rain that blew into the front of the shelter. Our front-row seats for the fire show weren't suitable for sleeping. Wet feathers were for ducks not hikers. A wet down-filled bag loses most of its insulating capacity, a disaster in the mountains. Without a sunny day, which was unlikely, Brite and I would have to sleep it dry with our body heat.

The only bright spot on the horizon was the line of food bags hanging from the trees like miniature hot-air balloons. That morning at the breakfast table, talk was about snorers and mice. Nothing kind was said about either. While the snorers had hacked through our sleep, the mice had gnawed through some of the backpacks that had food or food residue inside. Brite and I escaped the onslaught with no physical damage. However, throughout the night, we both felt tiny feet scampering across our foreheads. That was enough to cause concern. Shelter mice can carry Hantavirus, a potentially fatal respiratory disease caused by contaminated dust from mice droppings or nests.

Brite and I wobbled and hobbled for the first mile, still stiff and sore from yesterday's hike. In the cold rain, it took a few miles to warm up sore muscles, but once we broke a sweat, we didn't stop sweating. Our breathable lightweight Gore-Tex rain jackets didn't seem to breathe well and left us panting for air. Even though we were sweating freely under our jackets, we left them on for the warmth. We could change into dry clothes at the next shelter.

We strolled down the back side of Ramrock Mountain and crossed GA 60 at Woody Gap. Waiting on the other side was a welcoming party with a cooler of soft drinks and a box of candy bars—our first trail angels and trail magic. Among the crowd was a burly middle-aged man with a straggly beard, cradling a puppy in his arm, who looked like a cross between Santa Claus and Grizzly Adams, the legendary mountain man played by actor Dan Haggerty. The camouflaged floppy hat and the army field jacket over a flannel shirt and coveralls only enhanced the mountain image with a menacing edge. That notion was dispelled when I looked down and saw sandals with socks. *Maybe an old hippie leftover from Woodstock*, I thought.

Slowly stepping toward Brite and myself, our affable trail greeter introduced himself as Mark Jordan, former army ranger, outdoor photographer, life counselor, spiritual warrior, and Christian mystic. Following trail etiquette for the receipt of trail magic, we chitchatted. When I mentioned Herm's Hike, Mark stepped closer with a bemused look on his face.

"Are you a religious person?" he asked in a serious tone.

"I believe so," I replied, not knowing where the conversation was going.

"What religion, not that it makes a difference?"

"Old altar boy," I replied as we both laughed at the sobriquet for Roman Catholic. "How about yourself?"

"Believer in God and follower of Jesus Christ," he proudly proclaimed with a glint in his eye. "It's all a person needs to find their purpose in life."

"Not a bad religion at all," I agreed, nodding my head.

"One piece of advice, if I may? Out there," he said pointing to the trail, "you're alone with your thoughts. Between now and Katahdin, you're going to think every thought you had in your life at least ten thousand times. Embrace it, the good and bad. Your thoughts will lead to questions and your questions to answers. Seek and you shall find."

"Thanks for the advice. I'll give it some thought," I joked as we shook hands. I couldn't have agreed more with this Appalachian mystic. I had already thought about every thought in my life at least a hundred times. The trail was a time machine that was transporting me back to my childhood and college days through the good times and bad. At times, I spontaneously burst out laughing at some zany episode that miraculously surfaced from the past. Other times, I frowned when I remembered those I hurt and those who hurt me. Silently, I forgave and hoped I was forgiven for my lack of compassion.

After our break, Brite and I hiked up Big Cedar Mountain, our steepest climb to date. In minutes, we were wrapped in a cold blanket of suffocating fog. With visibility near zero, Brite and I literally vanished into thin air. To ensure that we didn't get separated, I took the cord from my food bag and rigged a safety line around our waists. Our only escape route was the well-worn path beneath our boots.

Heading down the mountain, the fog dissipated, but the rain turned into a steady downpour. The trail became a mudslide. Brite and I shortened our strides and leaned heavily on our hiking poles to maintain balance. Every step forward was half a step backward as our boots slipped in the mud. Each of us fell a few times, landing with a soft thud. To ease the pain of the ugly day, we sang every song we knew that had the word "rain" in the title or improvised lyric. Our singing only made it rain harder.

The death march to Woods Hole Shelter was twelve miles over inhospitable terrain. At around 4 o'clock, we arrived at the shelter to find that every inch of space had been claimed, to include the picnic table and the space underneath it. In the tent area, the situation was the same. There wasn't a foot of flat ground available. Brite and I looked at each dejectedly and frowned. The trail companion reported a campsite a half-mile farther up the trail. It was our only hope. Reluctantly, we slung our backpacks over our shoulders and headed back to the trail.

A half an hour later, we rested where the trail turned sharply to the right and uphill. A side trail to Bird

Gap was on the left. I searched frantically for a trail sign indicating the mileage to the campsite. Instinctively, I knew we were close, but there were no markers. To make matters worse, the landscape was fading into dusk.

"It's just over a mile to the shelter on Blood Mountain, but it's almost straight up the mountain. I don't have a clue where the campsite is located," I said haltingly as the rain streaked down the pages of my trail companion and map like teardrops.

"We need to stop real soon. My hip is hurting and I don't have too many more steps. You make the call," Brite replied wearily.

"Let's head down the side trail. There's got to be someplace to pitch the tent," I announced confidently, hoping to buoy Brite's sagging spirit. Hiking to the shelter wasn't a consideration. It was too risky to climb rocks in the rain and semi-darkness.

After a half-mile of treacherous loose rocks down the side of the mountain, we reached a primitive campsite that was flooded. The only level ground not underwater was next to the trail. Hastily clearing some brush, we hurriedly pitched Auntie Agnes about twenty feet from the bank of a small stream. Within minutes, we were snuggled in our sleeping bags, feeling safe and secure. Dinner was candy bars and gorp. With a good-night kiss, Brite seemed to have found her smile. It was the only bright spot of the day. We had hiked fourteen tough miles in brutal conditions. I just hoped that we hadn't pushed ourselves too hard physically. I didn't want a forgettable day to become a regrettable day.

Despite being totally exhausted, I tossed and turned in my mummy bag unable to fall asleep. In the howling wind and battering rain, our tent had become a lifeboat cast wildly upon a stormy sea. Other than the tent ripping apart or suddenly springing a leak, my biggest fear was that a tree would crash down on us like a broken mast on a tall ship.

Around midnight, I finally drifted off to sleep with the soothing sound of a rushing stream in my ears. The next time I opened my eyes, it was 4:45 a.m. With Brite sleeping soundly, there was no sense in getting up this early. It was dark and still raining, and the sleeping bag had dried to toasty warmth.

Staring into the impenetrable black void, I was already having second thoughts about the hike. *How could I live with myself if something happened to Brite?* I thought. To her credit, she was a trooper. Not a thru-hiker, she wanted to hike the first and last hundred miles to be part of this great adventure and pay tribute to my father. Although we were in reasonably good physical shape, I worried that we were in over our heads with long-distance hiking. A retirement vacation in the tropics seemed more inviting with each passing minute. With visions of sandy beaches and Brite by my side, I closed my eyes and drifted away on a cloud of doubt. Thankfully, I had doubt and not regret.

Finally at around 6 o'clock, we both stirred. "Did you hear it last night?" Brite asked sleepily.

"I heard it all, all night long, the rain, the wind, even some thunder," I replied nonchalantly.

"No, not that. I'm taking about the big swoosh," she exclaimed excitedly. "A tidal wave rumbling down the mountain. I was going to wake you when I first heard it, but I figured since I couldn't do anything about it, why bother. All I did was pray that we wouldn't be washed down the mountain in our sleeping bags."

Brite's tsunami story was amazing since I was the light sleeper in the family. At the slightest noise, my eyes rolled up like window shades. I wondered if her ears weren't playing tricks on her mind.

Inside the tent, we acrobatically dressed into cold, damp clothes that had been too wet to dry inside the sleeping bags. Our feet fared slightly better. Extra socks guaranteed dry feet for a few hours or a few miles.

Peeking out the tent flap, I cautiously surveyed our surroundings. The landscape was completely saturated. Although it had stopped raining, water was dripping off the trees as if they had sprung a leak. The ground was pockmarked with giant puddles. Now I knew how Noah and his shipmates felt when they stepped out of the ark after forty days of rain. Like me, they were just glad that it stopped raining.

Eager to reach civilization at Neel Gap, a mere four miles over the mountain, Brite and I exploded out of the tent to break camp amid a chorus of whoops and hollers. As we rolled up the tent, I noticed a snaking line of twigs, leaves, and stones only a few inches from the back wall.

"Holy Jesus, your prayers were answered," I yelled at Brite, pointing to the high-water mark from the stream.

"We're damn lucky for sure," she said as she came around back for a closer look. "I know a tidal wave when I hear one and I know one when I see it."

"Right as rain," I joked, making light of the near-disaster to boost our morale. Privately, I worried about our welfare. Our judgment had been impaired by exhaustion. We could have easily been severely injured or killed. I silently vowed never to let it happen again.

After retracing our steps up the trail, Brite and I discovered just how utterly frustrating the AT can be. At the trail junction, I finally found the weathered sign that pointed to the Slaughter Creek Campsite, a couple hundred feet up the trail. "Son of a bitch," we blurted out in unison with looks of disgust. We had hiked an extra mountain mile for nothing, not even a good night's sleep.

The hike to Blood Mountain, the tallest mountain in Georgia at 4,458 feet, featured steep switchbacks and rock scrambles. An hour later, we huffed and puffed our way to the doorstep of the shelter, a stone hut with a fireplace built in 1934 by the Civilian Conservation Corps. We took a quick tour to see what we missed. Nothing and everything! The rooms were dank and musty but dry, most likely with a large mouse population. We frowned in agreement and shook our heads. Anything indoors would have been better than last night's accommodation. We dropped our packs and walked around the shelter.

"You know what they need up here?" I said to Brite, who was nibbling around the edges of her Pop Tart that looked and probably tasted like Civil War hardtack.

"Other than a bed and breakfast, I wouldn't have a clue," she replied sarcastically, obviously her head still swimming from last night's aqua adventure.

"A totem pole," I exclaimed proudly. "Here we are in sacred mountains of the Cherokee, and most hikers don't have a clue about the history of this land. A totem pole would tell the story of the land and its people."

"I don't think they had totem poles. They had the alphabet. Letters are all you need to tell the story," Brite chided, laughing at her witticism.

"Then they need a bronze plaque to tell the story. What I need is to talk with a real-life Cherokee," I lamented.

"You have about as much chance of finding one as you do a sunny day," Brite grumbled dryly, now staring at her Pop Tart. Obviously, she wasn't interested in swallowing that or my comment.

Local legend reported that Blood Mountain took its name from a fierce battle fought between the Cherokee and Creek in the late 1600s when the mountain ran red with blood. To me, the mountain was more than a battle monument; it was a memorial to the Cherokee Nation and their spiritual legacy. The Cherokee revered one god, the Great Spirit who created Mother Earth. They believed that every function of life was connected. As long as man respected nature as an equal partner, the universe would be in harmony. Unbelievably, that sacred dogma of coexistence was a death sentence for the Cherokee at the hands of white settlers who believed that nature was to be conquered not cultivated.

In the fall of 1838, an estimated 13,000 Cherokee began their forced march west in what became known as the Trail of Tears. By the time they crossed the Mississippi River and reached Indian Territory in late winter, 4,000 to 6,000 Cherokee were dead from sickness, starvation, exhaustion, or exposure to the cold. Sadly, the march was a tragic prophecy for Native American tribes. The government's well-rehearsed script would be reenacted over the ensuing decades with the same results. Indigenous nations fell like dominoes to war and disease as the Manifest Destiny rolled across the country in wagons full of white settlers. For certain, I was going to need a large plaque for my historical project on the appropriately named Blood Mountain.

Chapter 3
Cheeseburgers for Jesus
(Neel Gap to Hiawassee, GA)

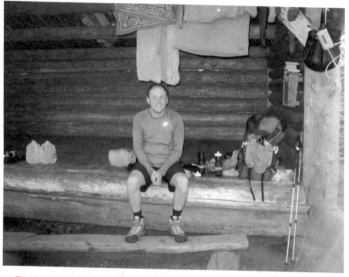

*Drying out my worldly possessions in the utilitarian AT shelter, a
frequent event.*

For the next two hours, Brite and I methodically picked our
way down the steep and rocky mountain trail. We learned
that gravity worked both ways. Going down was equally
as hard as going up, especially on the knees. I preferred
hiking up; Brite preferred hiking down. Together we were
a well-balanced hiking machine. Only a few hundred

yards from the highway, we suddenly stopped and sniffed the air like bloodhounds.

"Do you smell what I smell?" I asked Brite incredulously, not believing my nose.

"Hamburgers," she yelled deliriously. "Big, thick, juicy, greasy burgers on a grill."

"Must be a picnic nearby. Maybe we can yogi for some food," I hinted excitedly but cautiously, not wanting to get our hopes up too high. The practice, named after Yogi Bear (the picnic basket thieving bear from the kids cartoon show in the 1960s) was the good-natured effort by hikers to obtain food without asking. Once you asked, you were begging, and begging was against the ethical code of the thru-hiker. On the plus side, a hiker was only limited by imagination in developing a pitch or a ploy.

With the scent of sizzling meat in the air, Brite and I picked up the pace to Neel Gap. Crossing the highway, we spotted smoke billowing under the passageway at Mountain Crossings at Walasi-Yi, the former CCC structure that now housed an outdoors store. Volunteers were throwing thick patties of ground beef on a fiery grill. Our mouths watered as we approached the flames. "Food's served at eleven," someone yelled to the gathering crowd. It was only 10:15. Brite and I gulped hard and turned away.

To kill time, we took a self-guided tour of the store that was crammed with hiking and backpacking gear. We gawked at the hundreds of old hiking boots hanging from the rafters that represented epic stories of inspiration, perspiration, frustration, and exhilaration. Proprietor Winton Porter called the collection the "Old Sole" Museum. One day he hoped to have a pair of boots for each mile on the trail.

Outside on the patio, Brite and I joined the crowd for the daily backpack shakedown, also known as a "ruck tuck." At the cost of a few good-natured laughs, a hiker could lighten and lessen his load. After a backpack was weighed, a staff member from the store emptied its contents one item at a time with a running comical commentary. The "heavies" were usually extra clothing, cotton clothing, cookware, and foodstuffs, especially items in jars and cans. Some hikers literally did pack everything but the kitchen sink. "Go light or go home" was the mantra of the hour. After all, this was a mountain hike not a cruise vacation. Every ounce in the backpack was a pound on your back. Brite and I took mental notes.

Back at the grill, it was finally lunchtime. Our hamburger hostess was Suzy Miles, trail angel and official trail servant. While standing in line, Brite and I shared our story about Herm's Hike. After serving up our burgers, Suzy sat down and shared her story.

Growing up in nearby Dahlonega, she saw a void in the spiritual needs of hikers. In 2003, she and her husband, Miles, started the Appalachian Trail Servants to represent Christ through service, fellowship, evangelism, and discipleship on the AT.

"What about the hamburgers?" I asked Suzy, sensing more to her story. "Just trail magic for the sake of trail magic?"

"A divine appointment," she cheerfully answered. "We pray every day for a chance to share our faith and spread the gospel. We get that chance here at the trail crossing."

"Brite and I are divine appointments?" I queried.

"Yes, but especially you,' she replied boldly, looking in my direction. "Days or months down the trail, you'll see that it was no coincidence that you stopped for a burger. Walk with Christ and connect the dots."

Before leaving, I gave Suzy a Herm's Hike flyer and asked her to pray for us. She assured me that prayers from her church were forthcoming. I was tempted to calculate the membership of her congregation and make an entry in my trail journal under Prayer Credit. After last night's adventure, Brite and I needed all the prayers we could get. I wondered if Winton had any prayer cards for sale. He seemed to have everything else.

"By the way, Paul, what's your trail name?" Suzy asked before returning to the grill.

"Raindance," I sighed after explaining that Rain Man had been banned due to the weather. "I don't like it, but right now it's all I got."

"Don't worry, you'll get a better one. It's just one of the dots," she replied confidently. "Besides, I like Paul as in Paul on the road to Damascus. It has a nice biblical ring to it," she mused, looking up to the sky.

After gorging ourselves on hamburgers, Brite and I agreed that a good night's rest in a real bed would be the perfect way to end the day. With the store's hostel already full, I called Goose Creek Cabins, just three miles down the road. A shuttle would pick us up in fifteen minutes.

"There's your totem pole," Brite shouted, pointing to a highway historical marker that cited the battle of Blood Mountain and the Nunnehi, or "People Who Live Anywhere." The Nunnehi were a race of friendly spirit people who could take human form and speak. They often cared for lost hunters and wanderers in their great townhouses on the mountain before guiding them home.

"Sounds like a combination of trail angels and guardian angels," I replied. "Do you think they guided us last night to the stream?"

"No, they didn't guide us. They pulled our tent away from the stream," Brite replied with a hearty laugh.

As we waited in the parking lot with a small group of hikers also headed to Goose Creek Cabins, I spotted my trail guru. Mark Jordan was busy greeting hikers with his puppy cradled in his arm. He waved and walked toward us.

"How was last night?" he grinned.

"Like Noah's Ark in a tent," I replied, explaining our brush with a watery grave.

"Just one more piece of advice," he offered politely. "The AT is a journey of body and soul. Right now, you're a stranger in a strange land. Keep moving forward to the light. It will lead you out of the darkness to home." The AT mystic had spoken once again, and I was listening even if the message was cryptic.

As the van pulled up, I looked over at Brite and nudged my head in Mark's direction. "He is definitely one of the Nunnehi, no doubt about it."

"I couldn't agree more, especially since he's big enough to drag a tent," she chuckled.

Goose Creek was an answer to our prayers, a collection of comfortable rustic cabins next to a mountain stream. With friendly owners (Keith and Retter Bailey), shuttle service, laundry by the pound, and clean rooms with soft beds at a reasonable price, it was a hiker's paradise.

After hanging our tent on the back porch to dry

and bagging our clothes for the laundry, Brite and I indulged in hot showers to soothe our tormented bodies. With the thermostat on high, the one-room cabin quickly became a sauna. We craved heat as much as we craved food. The hotter, the better! While Brite opted for a short nap before dinner, I opted for a short walk. I needed some quiet time to clear my head and collect my thoughts about the first couple of days on the trail.

At the front desk, Keith confirmed my suspicion about the road in front of the motel. Brite and I had passed this way just a few days ago. The homestead of Byron Herbert Reece was about a half a mile down the highway. I wasn't going to miss the poet after all.

That afternoon I had the Reece farm to myself. I peeked in the house that was being renovated as a tourist attraction and walked the grounds. To my disappointment, Mulberry Hall, the shed where Reece did most of his writing, was currently being stored off-site. As a writer, I wanted to stand in the place where the great poet put his emotions on paper and to see the colors of Appalachia through his eyes.

Nicknamed "Hub" by friends, Reece was a quiet and humble man with a long frame and a long angular face. While caring for his parents who were dying from tuberculosis, he took a part-time teaching job at nearby Young Harris College. On June 3, 1958, suffering from depression and tuberculosis, Reece took his own life. The voice of Appalachia had been silenced, but his words would echo across the landscape forever.

Standing in the field between the house and the barn, it wasn't hard to picture Hub behind a mule and plow in the shadows of the mountains. Likewise, it wasn't hard to feel the sadness that hung over the farm. The hardscrabble farmer, who planted words and harvested rows of tender poetry in obscurity, deserved the recognition that eluded him in life. Heading back to the hostel, I hoped the Reece Society was successful in their restoration project.

The next morning, Brite and I were back at Neel Gap. Suzy and the AT Servants were busy setting up the grill and handing out snacks. We graciously accepted cookies, brownies, and a prayer before walking through the breezeway to the next white blaze. Climbing a stone stairway that led to the next mountain, the sun was finally shining to our sheer delight. We desperately wanted heat. But instead of heat, we got hot, real hot in a hurry. The sun quickly burned off the morning fog, and the temperature soared into the mid-70s. After three days of cold rain, we were hiking in the tropics where clouds of pestering gnats swarmed around our heads. All we could do was keep hiking and swatting along a rollercoaster of mountain gaps.

At Hog Pen Gap, we found trail magic from a trail-friendly family. This time it was a picnic with hamburgers, hot dogs, soda, beer, beans, potato salad, and folding chairs. A parade of hikers stopped for a quick bite and some words of encouragement. With good food and good conversation, Brite and I lingered. We only had four miles to the next shelter. Before continuing on the rollercoaster, we popped some Vitamin I (ibuprofen) for dessert.

Late that afternoon, we finally reached the blue blaze trail to the shelter and jettisoned our backpacks in complete exhaustion. The four miles of PUDs seemed like forty. I had to remind myself of the new time and distance formula for foot traffic. Luckily, there was no need to take another step. Next to the trail was a parcel of level and dry ground with campsites. After pitching the tent, we joined our neighbors in gathering firewood. That evening we dined around our first official campfire. Finally, we had a chance to talk with Gypsy, Flatlander, and B, hikers we had previously met for only a few minutes. It felt like a family reunion.

That evening Brite and I performed our daily physicals. Her hip pain was increasing, and my left ankle was aching from the numerous rollovers on the loose rocks. Small blisters were healing nicely. I went to sleep kicking myself for not bringing my soft ankle brace. It was in the back of the SUV.

The next morning, Brite and I celebrated Palm Sunday with a breakfast treat of hot oatmeal. After a couple of easy miles on the trail, the hiking turned to rock scrambling under a relentless sun. We countered with frequent water breaks and copious layers of sunscreen. Hiking down Blue Mountain, a 1,100-foot drop in a mile and a half, we reached Unicoi Gap to discover that we just missed trail magic of food and beverages. Off to the side of the road, we overheard a cluster of hikers animatedly debating the weather. We edged closer to eavesdrop.

According to the Blackberry, a severe weather front was headed our way. Tonight's temperatures were expected to dip into the low 30s with accumulating snow or freezing rain in the higher elevations. Without hesitating, Brite and I joined the group for a shuttle to the Hiawassee Inn. After our Appalachian tsunami, we were not going to tease Mother Nature and tempt fate again. Walasi-Yi had been an outpost; Hiawassee would be a base camp. It was time to wait out the weather. Two days ago, the weather was sponging; today it was sizzling; and tomorrow it would be snowing.

Chapter 4

Albert's White Lightnin'

(Hiawassee to Franklin, NC)

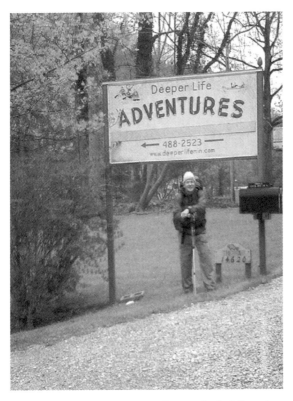

Sign outside the NOC that proved to be prophetic. More than white blazes pointed the way on a spiritual journey.

Located on the edge of town, the Hiawassee Inn was mobbed with hikers seeking shelter from the storm. To ensure that everyone got a room, the owner implemented a buddy system. Brite and I shared a room with B, the personable and savvy hiker from western Massachusetts.

That evening we dined with four other hikers at a family-style AYCE (all-you-can-eat) restaurant. I stuffed myself with slabs of roast beef and mountains of mashed potatoes with gravy. Even Brite, who had not eaten well for the last few days, had thankfully found her appetite. During dessert, it was decided to slackpack the next day from Unicoi Gap back to Hiawassee. With lighter packs holding the basic essentials, we hoped to hike seventeen miles before the storm arrived. Meanwhile, Brite decided to take a "zero" or off day.

At 8 o'clock the following morning as snowflakes fluttered in the air, we were shuttled to the trailhead. Two hours later, we were battling a raging blizzard that produced a whiteout on the windward side of the mountains. Winds gusting to forty-five miles an hour dropped the wind chill to the low teens. Despite the bone-chilling cold, I quickly broke a sweat trying to out hike the storm. Although my head and ears were covered with my knit hat, snow was stinging my face like blowing sand. Even with gloves, my fingers felt like icicles. When we stopped for a lunch on the leeward side of a mountain, I couldn't unzip my pack due to the numbness in my hands. Worse yet, I couldn't unzip my pants to go to the bathroom. All I could do was blow on my hands and wait for my fingers to thaw. Even my cold-cut sub was frozen solid. To eat, I broke off bite-sized pieces and stuffed them in my mouth to thaw. Most of the sandwich ended up on the grounds in frozen shards.

Back in town, Brite spent the day at the computer

catching up on family news. The good news was three contributions to Herm's Hike for $100 each. The bad news was that Brite was ending her hike. Her hip was hurting so badly that walking was painful. Instead of the 100-mile club, she would have to be content with the 50-mile club. There was no shame in that feat. She had hiked over fifty of the toughest miles on the trail.

That evening, Brite was despondent. "I quit before I reached my goal. I just plain quit," she said glumly.

"Nobody who comes out here with good intentions ever quits," I consoled gently. "It's just the mountains telling you to go home. When the mountains talk, you have to listen. It's that simple."

"Maybe you're right, but it still hurts. But one thing is certain, I'll be ready to hike again in Maryland and definitely in Maine, regardless of what the mountains have to say," she replied with a weak smile and tears in her eyes.

I was sad to lose my hiking partner but glad to see that Brite had finished the hike on her own terms. As a caregiver for my father, companion for my mother, business manager for Herm's Hike, and family administrator, she was the glue that held the hike together. Without her, Herm's Hike was over. The only consolation was that her injury didn't appear to be that serious. Now I only had to worry about myself.

The next morning all departures from the inn were canceled due to the weather. The tail end of the storm had stalled over the mountains, leaving the valley cloaked in a freezing rain and fog. While other hikers took advantage of the "zero" day to eat and sleep, Brite and I went to work. She headed back to the computer, and I headed to town to drum up business for Herm's Hike. Armed with a handful of flyers and business cards, I stopped at every church, nursing home, retirement community, radio station, newspaper, and public bulletin board that I could find.

At noon, I had an appointment with a reporter from the local newspaper. As expected, the reporter was polite and only marginally interested in my adventure. Only when I began to talk about my father's journey with Alzheimer's did he lean forward in his chair and begin to take notes. I had pushed the right button. My father's story was the key to opening doors. After taking my picture and wishing me luck, the reporter confided that several family members were battling the disease. With time on my hands, I crossed the highway to browse the Pick-a-Way Music Store and Pawn Shop.

"Hello! Anybody home?" I chimed as I entered the building. There was no response. Stepping lightly, I strolled down aisles of power tools, generators, snowblowers, and lawn mowers. Not much to look at since I already had enough tools back home to start my own pawnshop or hardware store.

What caught my eye were the rows of stringed instruments hanging from the ceiling. Mountain Crossings had boots and backpacks in the rafters. The Pick-a-Way had guitars, banjos, and mandolins waiting for a second chance at life. I recognized the names on the headstock, all of it top-of-the-line gear from Guild, Martin, Gibson, Fender, and Gretsch. I could have easily been standing in a pawnshop on Music Row in Nashville.

I stared in amazement at the collection. How many songs did they compose? How many honky-tonks, storefront churches, concert halls, and coffeehouses did they play? More importantly, how many broken, lost, and faded dreams did they witness? My imagination was in musical overdrive as I pictured Hank Williams with one of these guitars on stage at the Grand Ole Opry House. Suddenly, my daydream was shattered by a melodious voice from the rear of the building. "Can I help you, young man?" asked the elderly gentleman who had stepped behind the counter.

"Just killing some time," I replied.

"Well, I got the shotguns and rifles behind me," he joked. "If you're in no hurry, can I get you a cup of coffee?" he added after I introduced myself as hiker.

A minute later, Carol Underwood returned with two steaming cups of coffee. We sat and talked about my hike and his store. "You have an eye for quality. Do you pick any?" he asked expectantly.

"Played a little guitar in high school, but mostly the drums," I answered.

"Well, that's a real shame because I was hoping to play a little today. But no matter, grab your coffee and follow me. I think you'll enjoy this," he beckoned.

A few steps later, I was standing in the back row of the Pickin'-in-a-Holler, Hiawassee's answer to the Grand Ole Opry House. To my amazement, Carol had created a mini-concert hall in the adjacent garage bay. The backdrop for the stage was the façade of a country log cabin, complete with a porch and an awning.

Next to where we were standing was a small circle of folding chairs and guitar stands with an archtop electric guitar, an acoustic guitar, and an electric bass guitar. Carol picked up the archtop and began to strum some chords and pick a few notes. "Let's play some music," he said with a smile as he handed me the electric bass. "You're an old guitar player. Just follow me."

I plunked along with Carol for a couple of bluegrass and gospel songs as he strummed and sang. As we played, a handful of local musicians sat in for the lunchtime jam session before returning to work. At one time, the band had two acoustic guitars, electric guitar, banjo, fiddle, and bass. We were pickin' and a grinnin' for sure, playing notes that were as sweet and pure as a mountain stream.

Carol called it mountain music. He learned it from his daddy, who had lived and died in the shadows of the mountains. I recognized it as the music from my college days. There was no denying that the troubadours of late '60s and early '70s found their musical roots in the foothills and hollers of southern Appalachia.

As I was leaving, Carol announced to the small audience that I was hiking as a fundraiser for the Alzheimer's Association. Without a word, everyone reached for their wallets as he passed around an old baseball cap. "This is for your hike and your dad," he said sincerely, handing me $53 in small bills.

"I thank you from the bottom of my heart. I'm truly touched by your generosity to a stranger," I stammered, at a loss for words.

"No strangers here. Just a family of music lovers," Carol proclaimed cheerfully. "Besides, you're one of us now. You played the Pickin'-in-a Holler."

I gave Carol a flyer and a business card and invited everyone to follow the hike on my website. Heading for the door, I was stopped by a burly gentleman with a voice that rumbled like a freight train. "Paul," he said, placing his hand on my shoulder and looking me straight in the eye. "Last week, I had to put my wife, the love of my life for sixty years, in a nursing home because of Alzheimer's. My heart is broken. You're doing something very special here. I believe you're doing God's work. Just remember that failure is not an option."

Those final words echoed in my mind as I walked back to the motel. How would I define success or failure? Would it be money, miles, memories, magic, or miracles? Maybe it would be one, none, or all of these. Only time would tell, but how could you fail when doing God's work? I just hoped that God knew that I was on the time clock.

The next day I was back on the trail, and Brite was headed to Franklin to await my arrival. Despite slogging through slushy snow at the higher elevations, I had the best back-to-back days of the hike. The weather was sunny with intermittent showers and temperatures in the upper 50s. At around noon, I bagged my first state and entered North Carolina. One state down, thirteen to go, I mused as I joined James Taylor in singing "Carolina in My Mind." To celebrate this historic crossing, a trail angel had left a six-pack of beer and three miniature bottles of whiskey at the nearby campsite. While my fellow hikers reached for a brew, I grabbed the Bushmill's (Irish whiskey) and stashed it in my backpack. I had my triumphant toast for Mount Katahdin.

Ahead on the trail at the gnarled, ancient oak tree, I met Ancient Ruins, a retired police inspector from Scotland who had worked for Scotland Yard in London before pursuing a law enforcement career in Australia.

Like me, he was also living his childhood dream by hiking the AT. For the rest of the day, I enjoyed a treasure trove of "cops and robbers" stories delivered with a charming accent.

On paper the last day before Franklin promised to be rather easy, if there's such a thing on the AT. From the campsite at Betty Creek, the hike would be two miles over a thousand feet to the top of Albert Mountain and then ten miles downhill to Winding Stair Gap and a ride to town. About a mile up the mountain, Matchstick, my hiking partner for the day, and I noticed dark gray clouds rolling in from the southwest. We hurried our pace to get over the mountain and back into the woods. At worse, we would be in for a soaking.

About 500 feet from the summit, the hike turned into a rock climb. At certain points, we were clinging to the trail that seemed to go straight up the face of the mountain. Oblivious to the booming thunder and roaring wind that grew louder, we inched our way upward. Minutes later, we were hammered with a cold, numbing rain. With water rushing down the rocks, my hands and boots started to slip. I was slowly sliding backward when a deafening crack sent shivers down my spine. Jagged lightning bolts were stabbing the earth above us.

"We're in big trouble. Do you think we should turn around?" I screamed to Matchstick, who was about ten feet above me. At this point, I wasn't even sure we were on the trail.

"We'll never make it down in one piece. Let's keep climbing and make a run for it at the top," he yelled back defiantly.

His plan sounded foolish, but he was right.

Climbing up, we could see where we were going. Climbing down, we would be moving blindly on a slick surface. In that instant, I weighed my options and the odds. It seemed to be a matter of how I wanted to be remembered. I could either be struck by lightning or blown off the mountain. Certainly not the way I had envisioned ending the hike.

Looking down, Matchstick sensed my predicament. "Just follow me hand for hand and foot for foot," he yelled before making his first move. With a rush of adrenalin, I scrambled up the mountain like a hermit crab.

A few agonizing and frightening minutes later, we crested the mountain and sprinted across the peak. Foolishly, I slowed down to glance up at the fire tower next to the trail. A sharp crack shattered my gaze with a blinding flash. Plumes of smoke rose from the ground. My teeth rattled, my ears rang, and my whole body shuddered from the explosion. Momentarily stunned, I staggered for a few steps as the acrid smell of burning wood filled the air. The lightning bolt had split a large tree down the center about twenty yards behind the tower. Like an idiot, I had been standing next to a steel tower with two aluminum poles strapped to my backpack like a human lightning rod. So much for my vow to avoid compromising situations.

Gathering my wits, I turned and ran for my life. After finally catching up to Matchstick, we raced down the mountain, splashing the trail like frightened fish. Our biggest fear now was being blindsided by a wall of water from one of the feeder streams that crossed the trail. Fueled by a double shot of high-octane adrenalin, we ran until we collapsed by the side of the trail. By that time, we were safely down the mountain, thankful to be alive.

On the shuttle ride back to town, we were told that Albert Mountain was noted for fierce thunderstorms and lightning strikes. Most hikers that day had taken the blue-blazed trail around the mountain. Matchstick and I were among the handful of hikers who were at the wrong place at the wrong time and lived to tell about it.

Gazing out the window at the sullen day, I suddenly remembered that today was Good Friday. Surrendering to the old altar boy buried deep inside, I bowed my head and sat in silence, reflecting on the crucified Christ. I wondered if my prayer for this day had been answered or had I just been lucky, knowing that either way I was fortunate to be alive. Just then James Taylor's song "Fire and Rain" came to mind. Since the start of the hike, I'd seen fire and rain, but I hadn't seen any sunny days that would never end. I chuckled at the thought.

From the bus window, I saw Brite waiting in the parking lot of Ron Haven's Budget Inn with a worried look on her face. I immediately sensed that something had happened to my father. As I stepped out the door, she ran up with a huge hug and a lingering kiss. "There was a rumor that someone had been struck by lightning on Albert Mountain, and when you were late getting back …" she said teary eyed, her voice trailing off. When I told her about my hike up the mountain, I conveniently omitted the hair-raising details.

Much to my relief, Brite had three good days in Franklin. She called our daughters and my mother with updates, conducted Herm's Hike business that included stops at two local newspapers, and helped at the front desk of the motel. As an unofficial member of Ron's staff,

Brite gained access to all of the hiking scuttlebutt. The trail was taking an unusual early toll. A high number of hikers had ended their hikes in Franklin due to serious foot, ankle, and knee injuries that included breaks, bad sprains, and cartilage tears.

With hiking stories abound, Brite had one that was better than my harrowing escape from Albert Mountain. While using one of the motel's computers, she was joined by a female hiker with the trail name Aliyah. Given to her by a hiker from Israel, the Hebrew word had a special significance for its new owner. In a spiritual context, it meant one who ascends to a higher spiritual level. Nothing could have been more appropriate.

In his early sixties, Aliyah's husband had developed Alzheimer's disease. After years as the primary caregiver, she was spiritually, physically, and emotionally exhausted. Urged by friends and family to take time off, she regained her physical strength, but her spiritual health remained in a downward spiral. She defiantly questioned the existence of God and her purpose in life. Searching for answers, she explored religions other than Christianity, such as Native American, Buddhism, and Hinduism.

Borrowing dogma from each, she was finally able to comfort her broken heart with the understanding that a compassionate God does exist and that her experience with Alzheimer's was an ordeal by fire to temper the core of her soul. She could no longer dwell on the past because it no longer existed. She had to move forward with her life even though the steps would be emotionally painful. As a sign of her spiritual rebirth, she had taken off her wedding ring before starting the hike and prayed daily that her husband would pass safely into the hereafter, wherever and whatever it may be. No matter what happened on or off the trail, she would not be returning home for one year.

Aliyah and I had a lot in common. We were at the point in life where we had to surrender our ego (the selfishness of our vices) to the spirit (the selflessness of our virtues). Moving forward meant putting one foot in front of the other until we ran out of steps, white blazes, or pain. On and off the trail, we were passing through the shadows from darkness to light. To my disappointment, I never had the chance to meet Aliyah. I checked the shelter logs to no avail. If not on the trail, I hoped and prayed that she was still moving forward in some manner.

On Saturday, we had a catch'em-if-you-can pancake breakfast in the basement of the First Baptist Church. Suzy and the AT trail servants were standing by the door to greet hikers. After breakfast, Brite and I had individual and group pictures taken by a church member. On our way out the door, we signed the banner for the AT Class of 2009.

"God's work is never done, and God's grill is never closed on the AT," I joked to Suzy as we left.

"We travel the trail point to point. You have to connect the dots," she playfully reminded me.

That evening Brite and I celebrated our last night together with a gourmet dinner in the most unlikely of places. Our destination in downtown Franklin was the Café REL, a French bistro that shared space with a gas station. Entering the doors, we were transported to a Parisian café with the smell of freshly baked bread and freshly brewed coffee. Taking its name from the owner's initials, chef Richard E. Long, the bistro served upscale

French cuisine at peasant prices.

The following morning, Ron, the barrel-chested former professional wrestler turned AT innkeeper and entrepreneur, drove hikers back to the trail in his yellow school bus. Before boarding, I pulled Ron aside and thanked him for his hospitality toward Brite. I wasn't surprised by his actions. When I called him about shuttles to Springer Mountain months earlier, he reassured me, "Paul, just get yourself down here and we'll take care of the rest." He was a man of his word, a true friend of the hikers. When he announced the weather forecast calling for sunny skies and temperatures near 60, a chorus of cheers erupted that rocked the bus. Spirits were soaring with a palpable sense of excitement. For the time being, we were warm, dry, nourished, and resupplied. On this Easter morning, we were resurrected like the risen Christ. How could we not be happy! We had tenaciously survived our first week in Mother Nature's boot camp.

Chapter 5
To B or Not to B
(Franklin to Clingmans Dome, TN)

Ron's weather forecast was accurate. With high temperatures in the mid-60s, I hiked for the first time in shorts and a t-shirt. Although the few ounces of weight transferred to the backpack, I felt lighter and faster. I was grasping the mental game of the trail.

The trail in the Nantahala National Forest featured 4,000-foot gaps and 5,000-foot peaks. For the first time, I encountered a string of balds, large grassy areas on top of the mountains. Their origins have mystified scientists since colonial times because scientific data indicated there should be trees like those on the surrounding peaks. Lightning was one plausible theory, an explanation rooted in religion and science.

Cherokee legend told the story of a monster bird that swooped down and snatched children from their villages, never to be seen again. Answering the pleas of his people, the Great Spirit sent down lightning to destroy the monster and then decreed that certain mountaintops would stay bald so people could see danger approaching.

I clearly saw the connection. If Albert Mountain had been cleared, I would have seen the approaching storm in time to take cover. Regardless of what one believed, there was more science than science fiction in the legends of the Cherokee.

My hiking partner for the next two days was B, the roommate from Hiawassee. An attractive, very hip, and very strong hiker, she, like myself, was part of the Woodstock generation. While hiking, we often played "name that tune" for songs from the 60s and 70s. When I first asked about her trail name, the answer came in a song. "I gotta be me. I gotta be free. Daring to try, to do it or die. I gotta be me," she crooned.

"Sammy Davis Jr.," I bellowed when she finished, clanging my hiking poles together in applause. After a minute of walking in silence and musing about her trail name, I achieved a revelation of sorts. "B, you just gotta be. I think that's why all of us are out here. We just gotta be something and be somewhere, and at this juncture of our lives, it happens to be here on the AT," I intoned philosophically.

"To be or not to be is not the question, but the answer for us," she joked in earnest. We both shared a hearty laugh. As baby boomers approaching our "golden years," most of the questions about our lives had been answered. For mystic voyagers like myself, the trail was the logical place to find answers for those remaining questions about the meaning and mystery of life. I was writing the epilogue to my life while the younger hikers were working on the first chapter. If only I could turn back the clock, what would I do differently? That was food for thought to last at least two or three thru-hikes.

That first afternoon, I gathered with fellow hikers at the Wayah Bald Fire Tower for an extended rest break.

Built in 1937 by the CCC as a fire station, the stone structure was now an observation tower for tourists. On this gorgeous spring day, I viewed the bluish tint of the Great Smoky Mountains to the north and the green ridges of the Georgia mountains to the south. At nearly 5,000 feet in elevation, I was riding the crest of a mountain wave in an ocean of waves that melted into the horizon. The mountain surf was up.

With over a hundred miles of trail behind me and no longer a trail hodad, I was stoked. In my mind, I could hear the surf-pop duo of Jan and Dean singing "Ride the Wild Surf" and the Beach Boys singing "Catch a Wave." In some crazy way, I was fulfilling my pubescent dream of becoming a California surfer by mountain surfing. "Cowabunga, dudes and dudettes, I'm on safari to stay, shooting the curl in the heavies," I shouted at the mountains as bewildered day-trippers stared. After taking a few pictures of the set, I shouldered my backpacks and disappeared down the trail, leaving space on the crest for the next group of mountain surfers to catch a wave. I left my imaginary surfboard leaning against the tower rail.

A few miles down the trail, I stopped dead in my tracks. There was no mistaking the din of thundering hooves. Staring through the trees, I saw two riders galloping along a logging road when they suddenly pulled hard on the reins and brought their horses to an abrupt stop with loud whinnies. Voices drifted down the trail. I instantly recognized the female as B. Inching closer in a crouch, I clearly heard the Carolina cowboys, dressed in Stetsons and dusters, hitting on B.

"We have a cabin down the road. We can give you a hot meal and a warm bed for the night, or maybe it's a warm meal and a hot bed," one of the riders boasted with a southern drawl.

"I'm waiting for some friends to show up in a minute or two," B replied calmly. Seconds later, I rushed out of the woods to rescue a damsel in distress. I stood by B's side and tried to strike up a conversation with the men, but they were more interested in B than me.

"How about we share a drink, one for the road?" the other rider snickered, reaching for his canteen. "Right here, I've got some of the finest moonshine in the county."

B politely begged off, but I was game. Hoping this gesture of friendship would hasten their departure, I handed over an empty water bottle. "Just a sip will do for starters," the cowboy warned as I slowly raised the bottle to my lips and hesitated, a little leery that I could go blind from drinking homemade hooch.

"Sweet blindness," I yelled with delight as the sweet liquid trickled down my throat. "Sure doesn't burn like whiskey."

"That's real White Lightning, son. Nothing special in these parts," the cowboy bragged.

After the taste test, B and I quickly shouldered our backpacks. The canteen cowboy continued to fire questions at B about female hikers on the AT, but she ignored them. "What makes you so goddamn high and mighty that you think you can finish the trail?" he bellowed angrily, obviously frustrated by his spurned advances.

Before B could answer, I interrupted with my best imitation of John Wayne. "Fellas, this is one tough lady you're looking at here. Hell, I bet she could outride and outdrink both of you. If she says she can do it, consider it done." Without another word, the rodeo clowns shucked their reins and disappeared up the road. "Hi-yo Silver, away," I shouted.

"Happy trails until we never meet again. You creeps," B sneered.

That evening at the shelter, B and I shared our moonshine story at the campfire. We jokingly called it *Deliverance* meets *Thunder Road*, two popular movies about southern Appalachia culture. As the fire slowly died and the chatter faded, B surprised everyone and finally shared her life story.

In the late '60s, she attended one of the "Fame" high schools in New York where future artists and musicians honed their craft. Getting caught up in the social scene of the '60s, she did the "hippie thing" and spent more time at Central Park than in the classroom. Seeking direction, she decided to pursue a medical career. As a result, a nurse was born and an artist delayed. After fifteen years as ICU/CCU nurse, she sought a less stressful work environment and returned to school for a degree in fine arts.

Escaping to the Berkshires, she dusted off her nursing license and began working at a health spa/ wellness center while pursuing her art. Hiking the AT was a celebration of her rebirth as an artist. No one was more committed. She had rented her house to a summer theater group and could not return home until early September. It was a fascinating story. Heading back to my tent, Helen Reddy was belting out "I am Woman" in my head. I knew exactly whom she was singing about. B was a strong and invincible celebration of life.

There was another good story the next morning at breakfast. Wayah Shelter had been built in memory of two thru-hikers, Ann (Annie) and Larry McDuff (The Salesman), who were killed in similar bicycling accidents near their home in Alabama. After Ann was killed in February 2003, Larry raised over $10,000 to build a shelter in her memory. Sadly, he never saw his dream come true as he was killed in June 2005.

They enjoyed hiking, biking, and doing things together, much like Brite and myself. As I left camp, I couldn't help but think about how fragile and unpredictable life could be. One thing was certain. I was certainly going to pay more attention to the names of the shelters. In many cases, they were more than three-sided wood structures. They were monuments to unheralded Appalachian memories.

After a steep climb to the Wesser Bald Observation Tower at 4,627 feet, I stumbled down the mountain in fog and a drizzle for six miles to the Nantahala Outdoor Center, the whitewater mecca commonly known as the NOC. After the long descent, my kneecaps felt like sandpaper with bone grinding against bone. I quickly crossed the street, threw off my backpack, and reached for some Vitamin I. While waiting for relief, I found a comfortable seat on a wall overlooking the river and watched a handful of whitewater kayakers practice their maneuvers. Today's hike was done. I needed to rest. All I could do now was wait for the next hiker to appear and decide my next move.

A few minutes later, I spotted B walking across the footbridge from the other side of the river with a frustrated look. "Heading south now?" I joked. There was nothing funny from the look on her face. She was returning from the Nantahala hostel, an inexpensive cinder-block building that had bunk beds with no sheets or pillows. After hiking down the mountain, she had hoped for something a little more luxurious. So had I.

Due to the influx of hikers and kayakers, our options were limited. The local outfitter recommended the Nantahala Log Cabin Lodge just a few miles outside of town. Located on a steep hill overlooking the river, the ten-room lodge featured TV, refrigerator, microwave, coffee maker, and two queen beds at off-season rates. B made the call and we hitched a ride down the road. Minutes later, we opened the door to a rustic suite with a lofted ceiling and cedar-planked walls. After a week of stale, musty hikers and shelters, the sweet smell was an intoxicating, heavenly incense. Maybe I needed to carry a few cedar chips in my backpack.

After dinner at the River's End Restaurant overlooking the river, B and I returned to the lodge for a good night's sleep far from the maddening crowd. Minutes after the lights went out, male and female voices penetrated the wall, a deadly combination for anyone expecting a quiet night. I had my earplugs, but this was not a shelter. I had paid for peace and quiet and that's what I was going to get. As B and I discussed our options, the voices moved to the outside porch. "Not a good sign. There could be an all-night party right outside our door," I said exasperated. "I'm going to try and nip this in the bud."

Stepping outside, my worst fears were confirmed. Three men and two women were milling outside the adjacent room with beers in hand and wetsuits hanging from the rail. One of the men was cradling a guitar with a harmonica holder around his neck. It was worse than expected. The last thing in world I wanted to hear was a Bob Dylan wannabe, but fortunately I was haste in my rush to judgment. To my delight, I got a Neil Young wannabe instead.

My neighbors were white-water guides in their late teens and early twenties from Canada. They came to the NOC this time every year (the rivers in Canada were still frozen) for whitewater training and certification. Without too much prying, they said they were just having a couple of beers before bedtime. They had to be on the river at sunrise so the heavy partying would have to wait a couple of days.

"Hey, mate, how 'bout a nightcap?" one of my new neighbors asked. "We brought our own supply of Molson and LaBatt."

"I certainly can't be unsociable to our Canadian cousins," I declared. "As long as you keep playing, I'll keep drinking." One nightcap quickly turned into two before the mini-concert ended. An hour after stepping on the porch, I was back in bed sound asleep in the still of the night.

Morning brought a beautiful spring day and a good omen across the street from the lodge. There I stopped to have my picture taken under the Deeper Life Adventures sign at the entrance to the Christian campground. It was more than a sign; it was an auspicious harbinger. However, my good fortune was short lived. Minutes later, while crossing the railroad tracks just north of the NOC, I rolled an ankle on a loose rock. Crashing to the ground under the weight of my backpack, I screamed in pain. After a few seconds of writhing on the ground, I slowly rose with the help of B and gained my composure.

With no ominous sounds of tearing or crunching, I was somewhat relieved.

My "spaghetti" ankle had been a chronic problem since I nearly broke it while playing softball when I was twenty-one. The diagnosis was third-degree ankle sprain. I was on crutches for two weeks while recovering. The instability of the ankle was the reason that I wore high-top hiking boots. With the ligaments permanently stretched, each subsequent roll or sprain usually resulted in minimal damage. Usually, I only had to suffer a few hours or days of discomfort while still ambulatory.

"Damn it. You dumb son of a bitch," I muttered as I tried to walk off the pain. My ankle brace was now in Maryland. I hobbled back to the outfitter and bought the last elastic ankle brace and popped some Vitamin I. Luck was on my side because the first part of the day's hike was eight miles uphill over 3,300 feet in elevation to Cheoah Bald. On a bum ankle, I found it easier to go up rather than down.

After a night of massaging my ankle at the shelter, I reached Fontana Dam in mid-afternoon. With the Fontana Hilton (the name given to the spacious shelter with access to water, showers, and a pay phone) already full, I decided to spend the night with B and some other hikers at Fontana Village, a nearby mountain resort. My first order of business before eating and sleeping was to call home for any updates. After two tough days on the trail, I was ready to hear Brite's cheery voice with good news about anything.

"The FBI was at the house this morning looking for you," Brite said nervously and haltingly. "You're wanted as a domestic terrorist. They wanted to search the house for weapons and explosives, but I told them to get a search warrant. You have to come home right away. They want to talk to you as soon as possible."

"Those rotten bastards. They're coming after me with a vengeance," I fumed, exhaling a deep breath in disbelief. As a whistleblower against my employer for financial fraud and abuse, I thought I was out of reach because of my pending retirement. I had never been more wrong about something in my life. The long arm of military industrial complex was reaching out nearly a thousand miles to strangle me.

"You also received three certified letters from your command," Brite added solemnly. "One telling you that your security clearance has been suspended; one telling you to report to work next week or be dismissed for abandoning your position; and, get this, one telling you that you're barred from entering the post."

"How in the hell am I supposed to report to work if I can't enter the building?" I roared in frustration. "Call Neil (our lawyer) and get me an appointment. In the meantime, I'm heading home."

B was shocked and scared when I told why I was heading back to the trail at dawn. I couldn't blame her. For all she knew, I could be a spy or a serial killer. "Go home and take care of business. Hopefully, we can meet up in Hot Springs. If not there, definitely somewhere else on the trail," she said with a concerned look and a weak smile.

Unable to get a ride to Gatlinburg, I decided to hike to Newfound Gap and hitch a ride to Gatlinburg. From there, I would figure out how to get home. After spending most of the night either pacing the floor and staring at the ceiling, I gave up on sleep and shouldered the backpack. At 5 a.m., I walked across the crown of Fontana Dam, my thoughts focused on home. "A bridge over troubled water," I chuckled to myself as I enjoyed the view atop the 480-foot-high concrete monolith in the dawn's early light. That would be my last laugh for the next week. Despite the maelstrom that was waiting for me, I couldn't help but worry about Brite. When the two agents appeared at my door, she thought that I had been killed on the trail.

That day I hiked sixteen tough miles in the Great Smoky Mountains National Park on adrenaline and anger. At Spence Field Shelter I stopped for the night physically and emotionally drained. Unable to eat, I unrolled by sleeping pad and bag and collapsed in a deep, dreamless slumber.

At dawn the next morning, I was the first person out of the shelter for another sixteen-mile marathon hike to Clingmans Dome. Once again, my thoughts were preoccupied on my interview with the FBI. I had no doubt that knowledge of the cover-up had reached the highest link in the chain of command. Since the Vietnam War, the cover-up had become the army's tactical trademark. Any scandal that would jeopardize a high-ranking career would never see the light of truth, whatever the cost. In my case, the "green suits," the military staff, were eyeing lateral high-paying civilian jobs. They were determined to protect their turf at all costs. I had underestimated their cunning.

Hiking over an undulating ridgeline at over 5,000 feet in elevation, speckled black and gray clouds, filled with moisture, hovered low in the sky. As the day progressed, the rain fell harder and the temperature began to drop. I could now see my breath with every step. I was chugging and wheezing along the trail like a steam engine. Although soaked to my skin from sweat, my jacket was preserving body heat and preventing hypothermia. "Thank God and Gore-Tex," I mumbled.

Chapter 6
An Angel Appeared and Said ...
(Clingmans Dome to Parkton, MD)

In late afternoon, I arrived wet and weary at Double Spring Gap Shelter, the last stop on the way to Clingmans Dome. The place was crowded with raucous hikers waiting out the storm. Most of them were already snuggled in sleeping bags and talking about the next cheeseburger in Gatlinburg. I threw off the backpack and fished out two energy bars.

"Anybody heading up to the Dome?" I asked hopefully.

"We're waiting until tomorrow morning. The weather is supposed to break sometime tonight," responded a hiker whom I recognized from earlier on the trail. "It might be best to stay here and hike with us tomorrow. We've still got some room."

"I wish I could, but I have to get into Gatlinburg as soon as possible for a family emergency. I might have to get off the trail for a day or two," I said solemnly between gulps of water.

"Good luck, man. Hope it all works out whatever it is. Hey, see you down the trail. First round's on me," the hiker added, obviously seeing the worried look on my face.

I shouldered my backpack and quickly departed. I still had to climb 1,140 feet over 2.5 miles. Outside the weather was worsening and so was my physical condition. To stay warm, I hiked with my gloves and knit hat, but the cold permeated my skin as the altitude increased and the temperature plummeted. I was feeling like a human icicle. Halfway to the summit, I hit the wall. I barely had enough energy to lift my foot and take another step. All I wanted to do was curl up on the trail and sleep. Instead I dropped to my knees and rolled over on my backpack into a sitting position to rest. I had experienced glycogen depletion while running marathons but had never bonked this badly. I knew that I was in trouble.

Sitting in the trail, I assessed my situation. By my best estimate, I was halfway between the rock and the hard place, the rock being Clingmans Dome and the hard place being the Double Spring Gap Shelter. It was about a mile uphill to the summit or two miles back downhill to the shelter. I looked at my watch. It was 3:26 p.m. Under the current conditions, one mile seemed better than two.

I slowly rose from the ground and staggered forward. "Lord, you pick 'em up and I'll put 'em down," I groaned, incessantly reciting the hiker's prayer. A hundred yards or so later, I again fell to the ground to rest. Slowly rising, I now chanted the hiker's prayer aloud like a Buddhist mantra. Another hundred yards up the trail, I again crumpled to the ground.

"Lord, I need some help here. I don't think I can make it without it," I cried out in despair, looking up to the heavens that were obliterated by swirling dark clouds. I barely had enough energy to lift my head much less stand. The heavy rain had turned into sleet, and the wind was pushing a blinding fog up the mountain. "Just fucking beautiful. It's getting better all the time," I muttered sarcastically under my breath. At the rate I was moving, I'd be lucky to reach the dome by nightfall if I ever reached it all.

Once again, I lifted my aching body and hiked, leaning heavily on poles and moving like I was a hundred years old. Instead of poles, I needed a walker. "Lord, I'm still waiting. Anything you can do will be greatly appreciated," I roared against the wind. After another fifty steps or so, I found a seat on a rock and wiggled out of the backpack. My fuel tank was empty. I barely had enough strength to lift the water bottle to my lips.

Leaning back, I watched the trees, the mountain, and the fog come alive in a hypnotizing kaleidoscope of green, gray, and white. The swirling colors danced around me like mad wisps of smoke. Mother Nature was directing a National Geographic Special, and I was in the cast on center stage. Starting to noticeably shiver, I closed my eyes. A gentle warmth caressed my face and bathed my body as I drifted off to sleep.

"Hypothermia," my brain screamed hysterically. Like waking from a nightmare, I bolted upright, my eyes wide open and my senses alert. I was shaking uncontrollably, drowsy, and soaked in rain and sweat, certain that I was freezing to death. I desperately needed to get warm but there was no place to pitch my tent on the rocky trail. I thought about digging out my sleeping bag but that would provide only temporary relief until it got wet. The only thing to do was keep moving, one step at a time, no matter how slow. Hopefully, I was close to the summit.

"Well, Lord, I'm still here. How about a helping hand for an old altar boy?" I humbly begged one more time in a raspy voice.

Reaching for my water bottle, I heard loose stones cascading above me. Hopefully, a deer and not a bear, was my panicked first thought. I turned my head to see a pair of legs next to where I was sitting. With my eyes bulging, I looked up in disbelief. The man appeared to be in his twenties, clean shaven with short hair. He was dressed in a long-sleeved athletic shirt, running pants, and a pair of low-cut trail shoes. That was it! No sweater, no jacket, no hat, no gloves, no water bottle, and no daypack. I shook my head and repeatedly blinked my eyes, quite certain I was hallucinating. Too startled to speak and embarrassed at my madman ravings, I stared at the stranger in silence.

"I heard you from above," he announced in a comforting tone. "You're almost there. Just put one foot in front of the other a little while longer."

"I'm out of energy and almost out of time. I don't think I can take another step," I replied wearily, summoning the courage to speak.

"Yeah, I know. Just have faith in yourself. You'll be fine. Everything will work out. Just don't stay in one place too long," the stranger implored.

"Yeah, faith for the fatigued," I groused sarcastically.

"Exactly. Now you'd better get moving before it gets dark," he admonished as he bounded down the trail and disappeared into the fog.

"What the hell is going on here?" I stammered. The only person that I had seen on the trail the whole day had suddenly vanished into thin air. I jumped to my feet and ran a few steps after him. "Where are you headed?" I shouted frantically into the white void.

"The same place you are," a voice replied a few seconds later.

"And where's that?" I asked excitedly, thinking I was mere steps or minutes from salvation, which translated into a ride to Gatlinburg.

"Home," replied the fading voice that echoed down the mountainside.

I walked back up the trail and shouldered my backpack. "What the hell just happened here?" I mumbled in disbelief. How did the stranger know I was going home? I never mentioned anything about going home. And where was this guy headed? There were no roads or trailheads in the direction he was traveling. I knew because I had just come from there, and "there" was a long way from nowhere. If there had been a shortcut or a blue blaze trail down the mountain, I would have taken it.

The mysterious hiker was right about distance. Thirty minutes and a quarter of a mile later, I approached what I presumed was the summit, or at least a level piece of ground. Due to the dense fog, it was impossible to tell exactly where I was. Stopping to rest, I noticed the dead silence. The wind and the rain had stopped. The only sound was my labored breathing.

The mountain had become a granite tomb, guarded by a forest of ghostly sentinels who watched my every move. The stately fir trees that once covered the mountain had been killed years ago by a sap-sucking insect. All that remained were the skeletons of bleached trunks and broken branches. *Was this the white of the Divine Light?* I thought. Any second I expected my phantom hiker to step out of the fog and lead me home. Perhaps, the stranger was no stranger at all but my guardian angel, called to duty in an earthly form.

I may not have been certain of my sanity, but I was certainly lost. There were numerous well-worn paths on the peak but no signs to point the way. With visibility about ten feet, finding a white blaze was virtually impossible. Finding the concrete observation tower was improbable, but it was my only hope. Crisscrossing the summit plateau like a blind man, I literally bumped into the base of the fifty-four-foot tower. I had reached the summit of Clingmans Dome, the highest point on the trail at 6,643 feet.

Dropping my pack, I scurried up the ramp to the top of the tower. On a clear day, you can see a hundred miles into seven states. Today, I saw only fog. Back on the ground, I briskly walked down the half-mile path to the parking lot. It was 4:30 in the afternoon and getting dark. My only hope was to hitch a ride to Gatlinburg with a straggling visitor. As feared, the parking lot was deserted. I didn't even know if the road to the summit was open.

Fortunately, the restrooms were open. The men's room was warm and dry. If I had to spend the night on the mountain, it would be home for the night. While standing in front of the hand dryer, which I ran continuously, I slowly peeled off my wet clothing. As I was slipping off my pants, I heard a vehicle in the parking lot. I quickly zipped up my pants, grabbed my jacket, and bolted for the door. Hopefully, a park ranger had come to my rescue.

At the far end of the parking lot, I spotted five

people standing near a dark blue passenger van. Off to the side, an older woman, whom I presumed to be the grandmother, was watching two adults and two children feed a flock of wild turkeys.

"Excuse me, I'm hiking the Appalachian Trail, but I have a family emergency and need to get off the mountain today. Do you think that you could give me a lift?" I asked the older woman gravely.

"Mister, I'd love too, but I'm just the driver. You're going to have to ask the people who hired me," she said, pointing to a man and woman standing behind the children.

I took a few steps forward for a better look and frowned. The man, who had a shaggy beard at the end of a boyish face, was wearing a straw hat, a plain white shirt, and dark pants with suspenders. The woman was dressed in a plain, long cotton dress and a white bonnet. They were an Amish family on vacation. "Are they Good Samaritans, willing to help someone in need?" I whispered to the driver.

"They can be easily intimated by outsiders, but most of them are reasonable," she replied. Having lived in Lancaster County, Pennsylvania, I was familiar with Amish culture. I knew my chances were not good.

The gentleman listened attentively to my story without a word. When I finished, he rubbed his chin with his fingers and inspected me from top to bottom before stepping away to confer with his wife. From their facial expressions, it did not look promising. The man patted his heart and nodded to his wife before returning.

"We'll take you into town on three conditions," he said with a slight German accent. "It has to be good with the driver. You will sit in the front passenger seat and not talk to the children. And we will stop at the scenic overlooks on the way down."

"It's a deal. I just want to get to Gatlinburg this evening," I said eagerly. I ran back to the restroom and jammed the rest of my wet clothes into the backpack, wondering if my ride was a stroke of luck or the prophecy of the phantom hiker.

The ride around the far side of the mountain into Gatlinburg took about an hour and a half. There were a lot of pictures to be taken at the overlooks as the fog dissipated. From the van, I noticed the children stealing furtive glances in my direction whenever we stopped.

After a brief backseat conference with his family, the father asked me if I would be willing to answer questions from his children. Within minutes, I had them spellbound with tales from the trail like a modern-day Daniel Boone. They were amazed that people hiked over two thousand miles in the mountains and called it a vacation.

Entering Gatlinburg, the father instructed the driver to drop me off at the hikers' motel on the edge of town. As expected, he refused to take any money for his trouble. Instead of money, I quickly explained the moral code of the trail and thanked them for being such good trail angels. That brought a smile to everyone's face. "Good luck on your journey, Paul," the father intoned as we shook hands. "We will pray for you."

"You have touched my heart with your kindness. I can't thank you enough. You were truly a Godsend," I replied sincerely.

"No, Paul. We thank you for allowing us to bear witness to Jesus Christ and profess our faith as Good

Samaritans. And the children loved your stories about the trail. I think they would like to have you along for the rest of the vacation," he chuckled.

That evening the desk clerk at the motel arranged for a taxi ride in the morning. The nearest car rental office was at the Knoxville airport. Still frustrated and angry at the situation, all I could do was wait impatiently. In my modest room, I fell into bed and turned on the television, hoping that a mindless show would be the perfect sleeping pill.

After a few clicks on the remote, I found the story of Appalachia in a black-and-white documentary presented by the Ford Motor Company. Sleep would have to wait. The two-part program ran less than an hour but covered centuries of Appalachian life. The first part, *Children Must Learn* from 1940, was a condescending diatribe for government intervention to save the children of Appalachia from malnutrition and illiteracy. The "simple life" of the mountain people, as lovingly repeated by the narrator, was merely a code word for poverty. This was government doublespeak at its finest. I merely shook my head in disgust at the patronizing attitude, but that was the way of the world in the first half of the twentieth century. It was the same policy from the late 1800s, repackaged and gift wrapped for a new clientele. All the politicians did was substitute Appalachia for American Indian.

The second part of the show, *Southern Highlanders* from 1947, highlighted the culture of southern Appalachia. It was a fascinating look at the food, music, arts, and people. As the credits scrolled down the screen, I realized that while the trappings of Appalachian society had changed, the spirit of the people remained the same. Some of the people that I had met on the trail could have easily been portrayed in the show. Viewers wouldn't have known if it was 1947 or 2009.

The next morning I was on the road at daybreak to pick up my rental car. Wendy, my taxi driver, was a single mom in her late thirties who worked a number of odd jobs to keep the family financially afloat. Part-time hack, part-time bartender, and part-time seamstress to the country music stars who lived in the area, she had the wit and wisdom that came with a graduate degree from the School of Hard Knocks. Once the conversation shifted from her life to my current predicament, her van became a therapist's couch on wheels.

"My, my, this sounds like the Hatfields and McCoys, only instead of moonshine, you're talking money. It's got it all, power, greed, and corruption," she chortled. "Ain't nothing wrong in pointing out injustice. That's righteous. But whatever happens, make sure you walk away with your dignity. And don't forget to call me when you get back to Knoxville."

At 6 o'clock that evening, I walked through the front door of my house. At 10 o'clock the following morning, I was sitting in my lawyer's office. With my supervisor and the command staff conveniently out of the office for any of my phone calls, Neil was my only connection to the workplace.

My commander told Neil that he could not comment on my case since there was an ongoing investigation. However, he related that three of my coworkers had "voluntarily" come forward to say that I had vandalized government property, verbally assaulted employees, and threatened to blow up the office building. As a result of these allegations, the FBI was called to investigate me as a domestic terrorist.

For years, my agency had failed to comply with Office of Personnel Management regulations in regard to money for performance bonuses, mandatory overtime pay, and education benefits. Because upper management was military, they considered themselves above any civilian mandates. Any civilian employee who questioned their policies was sternly rebuked and reminded about job security. After a new civilian division chief looked into the matter at my request, she admitted that mistakes had been made in the past, but she couldn't correct the past. Since I was retiring, I decided to press the issue, thinking I was free from retaliation.

"Why would your coworkers make these allegations?" Neil asked with a befuddled look, unable to connect domestic terrorism with financial misconduct.

"Retaliation for requesting an investigation into the money matter," I replied dryly.

"But if you were retiring, that should have been exactly what they wanted. Once you were no longer affiliated, you had no redress," he opined.

"I don't believe they thought I was retiring. They thought I was trying to buy more time as my request for an official inquiry made its way up the chain of command. Last year, I had submitted my retirement paperwork to determine my eligibility, but I pulled the paperwork at the last minute."

"I've seen a number of smear campaigns against whistleblowers but never anything with so much malice. When I spoke to your commander he said that he would do everything in his power to see that you never set foot in the workplace again."

At high noon, the FBI agents from the joint antiterrorist task force appeared for the showdown that included an audiotaped interview and my sworn statement. The agents could ask me any questions as long as my lawyer could advise me whether or not to answer. As expected, the verbal sparring match began immediately when the agents refused to identify my accusers. Fortunately, an army official had inadvertently given the names to Neil. None of these employees had worked for me at the time of these allegations. Their stories were embellished third-person accounts.

Agent: Mr. Travers, three of your coworkers provided signed statements alleging acts of violence and terrorist threats by you in the workplace. Have you ever vandalized government property as acts of retaliation?

Me: No. However, on one occasion, I pried open my file cabinet with a screwdriver after a team member had accidentally locked all of the keys to individual cabinets inside my cabinet. The cabinet suffered some surface scratches and a minor dent to my recollection but remained in working condition.

Agent: Did you intentionally break a glass desktop in a fit of anger?

Me: No, but I did unintentionally break my glass desktop when I dropped a stack of files on top of the desk. The glass had already been cracked and was covered with scotch tape to prevent any further cracking.

Agent: Is it true that you threatened action against your superiors because you were denied a sabbatical?

Me: That's a ludicrous statement. I've been working for the government over thirty years. There is no such thing as sabbaticals for employees at my pay grade.

Agent: Did you threaten to blow up the building where you worked?

Me: No, but I joked in a private conversation that if Fort Meade was ground zero for a nuclear attack, our building would be the only one standing in the rubble.

Agent: Do you have any other comments regarding these allegations?

Me: If you check my personnel file, you'll find a spotless record, no reprimands, or complaints. Over the years, I received the highest performance ratings. Now let me ask you a question. I'm an honorably discharged veteran about to retire with a pension. Why in the world would I want to blow up a building and throw my life away?

Agent: That's what you have to answer.

Me: No. That's for my accusers to answer.

As the barrage of questions ended, Neil took center stage with the persona of Perry Mason. "Gentlemen, in light of my client's responses and his stellar career with the federal government, I believe you have been duped by an agency on a vendetta. I strongly suggest that you investigate my client's allegations against his employer."

After the agents left, Neil and I continued to talk. He thought I had a strong case for a defamation lawsuit. It would be the only way to bring the agency's misconduct to light. He was certain the money issue was only the tip of this malfeasance iceberg. On the downside, it would be costly and time consuming, and I would have to postpone official retirement.

"Neil, I just want to get on with my life and get back on the trail," I said assuredly. "If I pursue this, they'll have the investigation classified so no one can access it. The truth will never see the light of day. One man can't defeat an army of lawyers."

"I see your point, but next time see me before you blow any whistles," he remarked. "You handed yourself a death sentence by using your chain of command."

The following afternoon Neil reported that the FBI favorably closed my case. Also, he was informed by my command that no punitive action would be taken against me for misconduct if I agreed to retire immediately.

"Punitive action for seeking the truth. Don't you just love the system," I declared, flabbergasted at the arrogance of the military.

"But there is some good news," he added. "Your command has guaranteed your retirement paperwork will be expedited."

"How can they do that?" I asked.

"It's all in the stars," he chuckled. "Your case has the commanding general's interest." The top link in the chain of command had been rattled. The old adage about war had been proven wrong. Truth was not only the first casualty of war; it was also the last.

Chapter 7
A Patch of Heaven
(Parkton to Hot Springs, NC)

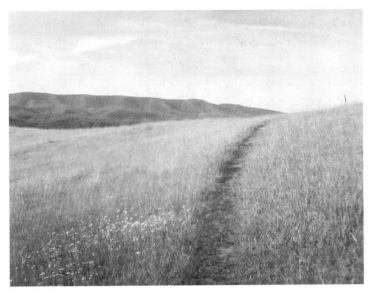

One of many balds in the south, always magical and mystical with breathtaking views.

When I suggested staying over the weekend, Brite jokingly grabbed my hand and led me to the front door. She saw the danger in a prolonged stay. I had to get back to the trail as soon as possible.

Late Wednesday afternoon, I changed into my hiking clothes, grabbed the car keys, and kissed Brite good-bye. My plan was to drive to Knoxville, spend the night at a motel, and catch my return taxi early the next morning.

The drive was boring and tiring with too much time to think. I simmered with anger at my former command and former colleagues, but that episode in my life was history. Now was the time to drop all the emotional baggage from my past and start living in the present. Where do I begin? Aliyah's story immediately came to mind. Maybe the answer was ahead on the trail. Hiking to Clingmans Dome had sucked every ounce of energy from my body and soul. It's no wonder that I was gasping for air. The breath of God that connected me to the universe had been completely expended. Who would breathe new life into my soul? As the miles rolled by, one nagging question remained: Who was the stranger on the summit?

The next morning at 7 o'clock sharp, Wendy was waiting outside the car rental office. "I can tell by the smile that things went well," she said cheerfully as I climbed into the van.

"What do you think?" I asked skeptically after giving her the rest of the story.

"Paul, you've got your pension and a ride back to the trail. I think that's a win-win situation. More importantly, you've now got your freedom. There are millions of people who would love to be in your place, including myself," she confided.

Two hours later, we arrived at Clingmans Dome parking lot. As I handed Wendy her fare with another sizable tip, she reached out and balled my hand in a fist.

"Sorry, but I can't take it," she said firmly. "I went

home and checked out your website. What I didn't tell you the other day was that my grandmama died from Alzheimer's. She was an inspiration in my life, the beacon of light in my darkest hours. I would crawl to Katahdin if it would bring her back for just one day. I want you to take the money as my contribution to Herm's Hike."

"Not even the tip?" I asked meekly.

"Not even. You're dealing with mountain women around here. We're strong, hard-working, caring, and, above all, proud. We say what we mean," she replied. I sheepishly placed the money back in my pocket. We hugged one more time with tears in our eyes. "Now get those chicken legs down the trail. You've got a lot of miles and money to make," she yelled out the window with a wave of her hand. I waved back and smiled as the van disappeared down the mountain. I just hoped nobody overheard her last comment. Chicken Legs wasn't my idea of a trail name.

Under a bright, blue sky. I quickly joined the tourist parade to the observation tower. At the top, I focused on the sea of rolling mountains to the north. They were the guideposts to lead me back home in two months. I closed my eyes and took a deep breath before slowly exhaling. Standing on that mountain, I felt reenergized. I was truly free. Wendy had a knack for saying the right things at the right time.

Back on the ground, I strode confidently into the woods. "Thank you, God. No help needed today," I shouted joyously. The day was shaping up to be a perfect prescription for the whistleblowin' blues.

Eight miles and about three and a half hours later, I crossed US 441 at Newfound Gap and stopped at the

Rockefeller Memorial. The Rockefeller Foundation had donated $5 million to buy land for the creation of the park. It was also the site where President Franklin D. Roosevelt dedicated the park on September 2, 1940. "Money well spent, gentlemen," I proclaimed jubilantly while taking a swig from my water bottle. As I was enjoying the scenery, I was approached by a retired couple on vacation.

"Thru-hiking?" the man asked kindly.

"For now, anyhow," I grinned with a nod of the head.

"Thought you might like a little treat to get you down the trail," he said, handing me a paper bag filled with two candy bars, two small pies, and two energy drinks.

"Dinner for two." I chuckled in appreciation of their kindness. "Too bad the Mrs. isn't here to enjoy it."

After a brief chat about my hike and a Q&A session, I thanked them and headed up the trail. I stopped and watched their car disappear down the road to Gatlinburg.

Typical of many road crossings, the parking lot had become a "hiking zoo" for tourists to gawk at hikers and daydream about their own thru-hike. Some hikers found the practice annoying, but I was flattered to be recognized as a mountain man. After all, it had been my childhood dream.

Back on the trail, I stopped to enjoy the stunning views from Charlie's Bunion. While on a hike in 1929, Charlie Conner and Horace Kephart, famed AT pioneer and noted outdoors writer, decided the rocky outcropping stuck out like the bunion on Charlie's foot. Like most quirky names on the trail, it stuck. However, I didn't see the resemblance.

Physically exhausted but mentally rejuvenated, I arrived at Peck's Corner Shelter Hours in the early evening. While digging out my sleeping bag, I found another of Brite's ubiquitous love notes that had been secreted away in my backpack and a flyer for a Bible summer camp titled "Paul's Dangerous Journey to Share the Truth." I didn't know where she had found the flyer but I loved her sense of humor. By 8 o'clock, I drifted off into a deep sleep with no second thoughts about returning to the trail. Brite had been right to boot me out the door. The trail was my home away from home, and it felt good to be back home again.

Back on the trail just after dawn, I realized the sun had missed its wake-up call. In its place, another storm front had settled over the mountains. The spectacular views on the ridgeline were shrouded in a soupy mix of fog and heavy drizzle. Determined to catch up with my tribe, I battled the elements to Davenport Gap Shelter.

The shelter, a stone dungeon with a chain-link fence at the entrance, was as depressing as the weather. Fencing, once a common feature at shelters, was removed after hikers began feeding bears from the inside. Although dark and dreary, the shelter was a dry place to rest my head. The Standing Bear Farm Hostel, a collection of buildings that resembled a hillbilly homestead, a hippie commune, or a combination of both, was only four miles ahead. It might as well have been forty. Long-distance hiking was not a game of inches and seconds like many sports, but a game of miles and hours. Today I still had a few hours but no more miles in my legs. The dungeon would be home for the night.

The next morning I hiked to the hostel for a

breakfast of hot pizza and hot coffee. After the perfect prescription for the Smoky Mountain Sunday mornin' blues, I headed to Max Patch Summit. Arriving at the expansive bald in late afternoon, I found myself surrounded by day hikers, day-trippers, and sunshine. I nodded and smiled at the sight. Some hikers were already busy illegally erecting tents for a memorable night on the summit. Not wanting to incur the wrath of any more federal officials (the property was administered by the US Forest Service), I hiked over the summit to a spot near the tree line where my gray tent would be perfectly camouflaged in the winter woods.

Back on the summit for dinner, Mother Nature treated her dinner guests to a spectacular show. As the wind increased in intensity, swirling alabaster clouds snaked their way around the nearby peaks and charged toward us like an army of ghosts. Our mountain view was obliterated. Seconds later, as if on cue, the curtain of clouds parted to reveal distant mountain peaks shimmering in sunlight. We sat in awe as the scene repeated itself two more times before the final curtain. After the last cloud retreated into the horizon, we jumped to our feet and applauded in unison. A standing ovation for Mother Nature was in order.

By the time I arrived at my campsite, dusk had turned to night. Changing into my silk pajama bottoms, I wiggled my way into my sleeping bag. After three days of hiking big miles in the big mountains, I was tired. Tomorrow there was only one mountain to Hot Springs. With the last ten miles of downhill hiking, visions of a soft mattress and a hot meal danced in my head. Hopefully, B and the others were still in town.

A little after 1 o'clock, I was awakened by the sounds of my tent straining against the wind. I opened my eyes and listened as the tent trembled. Outside, the wind hissed through the trees like ocean waves splashing on a sandy beach. Another storm was brewing. Before it arrived, I wanted to see the bald at night. Grabbing my headlight, jacket, and camp shoes, I crawled stealthily from my nylon cocoon.

Following the well-worn path to the summit, I tiptoed through the gypsy camp. At the edge of the bald, I faced east and extended my arms as if taking flight. My jacket flapped in the wind like an unfurled flag. Before me, an endless ocean of twinkling stars stretched to infinity. Staring at the heavens, I was quickly hypnotized by the night sky. *How many stars? How many planets? How many dreams had been pondered and plundered by mystic voyagers who dared to reach out and capture the magic of the light?* I pondered. Suddenly, there was a profound silence as deep as the night. The wind has taken its last breath.

At that moment, I heard a faint whisper from the darkness. "Be still and know that I am God," the voice commanded. I closed my eyes and instinctively fell to my knees, humbled by the power and glory of the unseen presence. Opening my eyes, I reached out to touch the heavens. A warm, tingling sensation radiated throughout my body as my fingertips disappeared into the inky edge of eternity. Time had stopped; my physical existence suspended. For a nanosecond, I was one in spirit with the universe, past, present, and future, and one with those who came before me and those who would follow.

A freshening wind, the divine breath, broke the spell. I slowly rose to my feet and continued to stare at the stars in wonderment. I said a prayer of thanks and retraced my steps. Once again snuggled in my feathered cocoon, I thought about the current journey of my loved ones back home until I fell asleep. I wished that I could be with them tonight. A second later, I realized that I had.

The hike to Hot Springs passed in a blur. I was light on my feet and even lighter in my heart. My soul had been drained and filled with a new energy. The vices of negativity (ego) had been replaced with the virtues of positivity (spirit). With each step, I performed a mental "ruck tuck" on my spiritual backpack. Now was the time to throw out any superfluous baggage and make room for more caring, compassion, and love. Throughout my life, I had carried the emotional flotsam of others. No longer would I live in their past and carry their burdens. There no longer was a past, only a present. The next step on the trail was the next step in my life. The mantra of "let go and let God" reverberated in the canyons of my mind. I was now certain that ancient mystics were the first disciples of the "go light or go home" backpacking mantra.

For much of the day, I was lost in thought about the mysteries of life. Last night on the bald, I became part of something greater than myself. I was one of those dots in heaven that connected to the infinity of the cosmos. One day, the timeless river that was the ever-expanding universe would ferry my soul to its outer edges where all of the secrets of life would be revealed. I would no longer be connected but united with the Creator. My transcendent moment on the mountain bald had not been a transformation but a revelation, one of the many that I hoped awaited me on my journey. *Just keep connecting the dots,* I thought. Suzy Miles was more than a trail angel;

she was a trail prophet.

Late that afternoon, I strode triumphantly into Hot Springs. Except for a few hikers, the trail town was largely deserted, a good sign if I was to find food and lodging. I followed the AT plaques embedded in the sidewalk and passed the visitors center. The "welcome" sign had been bulldozed and was leaning in a pile of rubble. "Not a good sign," I surmised.

After walking the length of the town, I headed to the Sunnybrook Inn, the legendary hostel owned by Elmer Hall. They were booked full. It was suggested that I try the Iron Horse Inn near the railroad tracks.

Retracing my steps to the edge of the town, I met a fellow hiker who told me that Flatlander was in Gatlinburg, B had gotten off the trail due to shin splints, and Gypsy had vanished. The Appalachian diaspora had begun. I no longer belonged to a tribe.

At the Iron Horse Station, I held the front door open for a group of partygoers who were headed for a waiting van. The last person to exit was a young lady with long brown hair who was clutching the arm of a friend. She walked rather stiff-limbed as if struggling to maintain her balance with each step. "So sorry," she apologized with a warm smile after bumping into me.

After checking in, I headed across the street to the Spring Creek Tavern. Pub grub and a few cold beers were the prefect elixir to celebrate another week on the trail. As I entered, a group of hikers that I recognized from Double Spring Gap Shelter waved me over to their table.

"Dude, we wondered what happen to you since no one had seen you in a week. We thought you quit and went home," said Mike, the bearded, burly hiker who suggested that I spend the night at the shelter.

"Went home and was resurrected is more like it," I replied. "Are you guys ready for the story?" They eagerly nodded their heads in agreement.

Over the first beer, I began to recount my experience as the FBI's "most wanted" thru-hiker as others sitting nearby joined the group. When I finished my life as a fugitive, they looked warily at each other with raised eyebrows. "The whole truth and nothing but the truth, my trail brothers and sisters," I exclaimed. Sensing their disbelief, I passed around the business card from one of the FBI agents. "Give him a call," I said defiantly.

After a toast to the newly minted folk hero who fought for truth, justice, and the American way of life, the conversation returned to the trail. When queried about their night at Double Spring Gap Shelter, my colleagues informed me that I was the last person they saw until they reached Clingmans Dome the following day. On the summit, no one matched the description of my guardian hiker. After the fourth free beer, I returned to my room, not knowing that it wouldn't be my last. My FBI story would become one of the longest beer runs in the history of the AT. It was good for a free beer in nearly every hostel and tavern from North Carolina to Maine. America certainly loved its outlaws.

The next morning before hitting the trail, I called home for any updates. "As of close of business on Friday, you were officially retired from the United States government," Brite chortled.

I laughed along with her. I was the recipient of a bureaucratic miracle. A process that took a minimum of sixty to ninety days had been completed in three. I was now retired with no rights, no recourse, and no retribution. All I had to show for my thirty years of processing security clearances was a monthly check. My new job title was long-distance hiker. Not having to punch a time clock for the rest of my life always brought a smile to my face. My challenge was now to live long and cash as many checks as possible.

Hoping to start the day with a fresh cup of coffee and a couple of doughnuts, I stopped at the Iron Horse coffee shop and gift shop. The door was locked. Peering in the window, a woman rushed from behind the counter. "We're not open yet, but come on in and get comfortable. I just started a fresh pot of coffee."

While sitting at the counter, Karen and I engaged in casual conversation about Hot Springs, Herm's Hike, and my father's plight in the nursing home.

"It should be one of Dante's inner circles of hell, yet it is a place filled with mystery and miracles," I began. "At the nursing home, I've met some patients whose everyday battle to live is truly inspiring. They have become my new heroes. Just yesterday, I saw a young handicapped lady leaving the restaurant with a smile that lit up the night."

"Long brown hair and wearing pink pajamas?" she asked with a bemused look.

"Yep," I replied. "And getting into a blue van."

"Why that was my daughter. Yesterday was her birthday," she exclaimed with surprise. "Now let me tell you my story," she said as she refilled my cup.

At the age of twenty-four, Jenna, just a couple years out of college and beginning a career, suffered a brain injury during a routine surgical procedure that left her in a life-threatening coma for over five months.

Doctors predicted she would be in a vegetative state for the rest of her life. Institutional care was recommended.

Vehemently disagreeing with the prognosis, Karen and her husband brought Jenna home to Hot Springs and began comprehensive therapy that included a therapeutic riding program. Her recovery in the saddle was nothing short of miraculous for improving motor skills, regaining strength, and restoring confidence in the will to live. After battling the hospital and insurance companies for years, a financial settlement was finally reached that would cover Jenna's health care for the rest of her life.

When Karen had finished her story, we both wiped tears from our eyes. "What a beautiful and heroic love story. You and your daughter are amazing people," I rasped, my emotions choking my throat.

The arrival of other customers signaled my departure. I posted my flyer on the bulletin board and headed out the door. Minutes later, I passed the entrance to the Hot Springs Resort and Spa. The mineral waters, first discovered by the Cherokee Indians, were noted for their healing powers. Too bad I couldn't stay longer. I would have loved a good soak, or maybe, the chance to heal.

Ascending into the mountains, I thought about Jenna and her courageous journey. Tears flowed freely down my cheeks as I thought about my daughters. I was truly blessed to be the father of two charming, intelligent, and compassionate women who were starting their adult lives. In the late '60s of my youth, they would best be described as "beautiful, hip, and groovy people." I liked that connotation.

In the back of my mind, a song was gushing forth.

Seconds later, I was once again softly singing with James Taylor. "Shower the people you love with love. Show them the way you feel. Things are gonna be much better if you only will," I crooned to the trees. The voice was definitely off-key, but I doubt if anyone had ever sung the song with more emotion. Sweet Baby James seemed to be shadowing me on the trail. He was good company for a walking man like myself.

High above the valley, I stopped at Lovers Leap Rock to enjoy the sweeping views of the countryside. Local lore told the story about the tragic death of Mist-on-the-Mountain, the daughter of Cherokee chief Lone Wolf. Near this spot, the beautiful maiden leaped to her death after witnessing the murder of her true love at the hands of a jealous rival. While the tale proved the power of love at any and all costs, the most powerful and prevailing love story was found in Hot Springs. And it didn't cost a thing. The story and the coffee were on the house.

Chapter 8
The Name Game
(Hot Springs to Erwin, TN)

Disaster struck the following morning at Little Laurel Shelter. While lunging over the picnic table to retrieve my falling Pop Tart, I heard a snap and a pop. I knew instantly what happened. Absentmindedly, I had placed my camera in my front pants pocket instead of the customary shoulder pouch on my backpack. Upon close inspection, there were no visible cracks in the casing or lens. I kept my fingers crossed and hoped for the best.

About a mile up the trail, I stopped at Camp Creek Bald, the first in a string of balds that extended seventy miles to Roan Mountain. In the early '70s, the bald was Viking Mountain, home to the Viking Mountain Ski Resort that had included Elvis as a guest. All that remained today were some ruins and a few roads. With the peak still retaining breathtaking views, it was time for some photos. The camera came to life with a rush of blinking lights and a low-battery warning. I replaced the batteries, took a few photos, and turned off the camera.

Ten miles up the trail, I stopped for more photos at the Civil War gravesites of William and David Shelton, both Union soldiers. On July 1, or sometime in early July

1863 (depending on the source), while returning home for a visit (either a family reunion or a recruitment trip, depending on the source), the brothers along with their nephew Milliard Haire, age thirteen, were ambushed by a Confederate raiding party, either on the road or at their cabin (depending on the source), and buried at this spot. They were gone but never forgotten. In 1915, a group of local pastors procured standard government headstones from the War Department for the brothers. Haire, a civilian, had to wait until 1994 for his marker that was donated by descendants.

I doubted that many hikers knew the historical significance of this final resting place. The war not only split the country but also divided southern Appalachia from the rest of the South. The Scots-Irish, who populated these mountains, had little empathy for the politics of plantation slave owners in the east while they scratched out a living as dirt farmers. Vitriol over states rights' and slavery often split mountain communities into opposing bands of armed guerillas. The Shelton gravestones marked the beginning of the Civil War along the AT. Once I reached the Shenandoah Valley in Virginia, I would be shadowing Lee's army north until it reached Gettysburg.

Turning on my camera, I was greeted by a rush of blinking lights and then nothing—no lights, no warning, and no power. The camera had drained the new batteries, and I had no more spares. Mental snapshots would have to suffice until I could purchase a new camera in Erwin forty miles up the trail. Any ideas of a photo album were on hold.

Two days later at Big Bald, an alpine bald at 5,516

feet, I met the motley crew from Spring Creek Tavern. The Spring Creek Gang, as I affectionately called them to their delight, had been reduced to a rugged and rowdy quartet. Big Mike, who had welcomed me at Double Spring Gap Shelter, had left the trail. As we chatted, a local hiker was regaling a circle of hikers with the history of the bald. Being a history buff, I couldn't resist. I dropped my pack and took a seat.

In the early 1800s, David Greer, nicknamed Hog, headed west from Asheville after a failed romance. With a rifle, a knapsack, and $250, he got as far as Big Bald Mountain. For the next thirty-one years, he lived as a hermit. Declaring himself a sovereign of the mountain, he harassed county officials about taxes and accosted trespassers at gunpoint. Ultimately, his confrontations with outsiders proved deadly when he killed a trespasser in cold blood. Found not guilty by reason of insanity, he was murdered months later in an act of revenge. But the end of his life was not the end of his story. During his exile on the mountain, Greer penned treatises on government and human development that reflected the ideology of the Transcendentalists. My interest was piqued. The hermit with the dark side was a humanist. Days later at a computer, I discovered that Greer was purported to have written the following:

"On arriving here on this lofty naked mountain-top and casting my gaze about, my heart began to heave and swell with strange sensations I have never before experienced. Look which way I would, Heaven, Earth and Ocean (the distant blue mountain horizon appearing as an ocean) seemed exhibited to my view in such a magnificent boundless prospect that my senses were bewildered and my mind filled with a dreadful thought of the Omnipotent power of a creative God! At length these overwhelming reflections seemed to nearly annihilate my personal identity and I felt as a mere atom of animate organism in the boundless universe."

A madman or hopeless romantic, it didn't matter. We were kindred spirits who shared mystical experiences on the balds. I couldn't have said it any better. While his long-forgotten words spoke volumes for me, I wouldn't have relished meeting Hog Greer on the trail.

By the time I arrived at the campsite Near Spivey Gap, the gang had set up their tents and started a fire. I quickly set up my tent, grabbed my food bag, and headed for the flames. As darkness descended, the sweet smell of burning marijuana filled the air. Clouds of marijuana smoke hovered overhead like hippie halos.

"Nah, man, I'll pass. I already did the '60s scene with Woodstock." I chuckled, waving off the pipe.

"No problem, man. Hike your own hike. I'm down with that," Recon replied lazily, already mellowing out. However, I did take a swig out of the flask that was being passed around. Burning its way to my stomach, the whiskey tasted good as it would to any mountain man. For some hikers, a nightcap of weed and whiskey was just another way to relax after a hard day on the trail.

As the gang and others found a comfortable spot around the fire, the idle chatter became louder and the trail stories funnier. Being the outsider in the group, I nodded, laughed, and occasionally asked a question to keep the story alive. After a few more hits on the flask, I stood to leave.

"Not so fast, old timer," Recon chided playfully.

"We checked your website to figure out this mystery man among us. Pretty impressive resume—author, Marine Corps officer, park ranger, and Herm's Hike—but we still don't know your trail name," he intoned as the gang murmured in agreement.

I had been outed. They were astounded that someone who had been on the trail for weeks didn't have a bona fide trail name. Justifiably I wouldn't be a legitimate member of the AT family until I had one. That moniker was your password to the AT culture and symbolic of your new life on the trail. Anything you did or wanted to do, the way you walked or talked, or what you liked or disliked was fair game for the name. The possibilities were limited by one's imagination. Normally you were given a name by fellow hikers, but it was just as acceptable to freelance your own badge of honor.

Recon, the outspoken and convivial leader of the gang, was an army veteran who had served a couple of tours in Iraq. Muffin, who appeared to be his current romantic interest, simply loved to eat muffins or so she said. Comments about her being a love muffin gave me second thoughts. Flipper had studied marine biology in college, and Tree was a genetic hodgepodge, a gangly young man with disproportionately long arms.

Under interrogation by my peers, I did what any nameless and shameless hiker would. I leaned back with my arms folded across my chest and began my woeful tale of anonymity.

Since I liked to walk in the rain, I named myself Rain Man, but there already was one from Nashville who made annual appearances as a section-hiker. After my impromptu rain dance failed to make it stop raining, I was tagged with Rain Dance. Being tired of the constant rain, I quickly discarded it. For a few days, I was Apostle, but I found that too pretentious in the Bible Belt, and there was already one from the previous year. Just Paul was just too plain. Grin, my college nickname for my ever-present smile (yes, life was good back then) made a brief appearance. That brought back a lot of great memories, but in reality, I didn't like any of them because they failed to reflect my rebirth on the trail.

When I had finished my soliloquy, Recon conferred in hushed tones with others. He stepped away from the fire and returned with a hiking pole in his hand.

"My noble band of brothers and sisters admire ye effort to honor thee father with thee hike," he announced with a bombastic English accent.

"Doth ye consider yourself the proverbial good son, wayfarer?"

"I like to think so. That's why I'm out here," I replied nonchalantly, not knowing what Recon had in mind.

"Then come hither, noble and loyal son of Herman," Recon commanded. "Kneel and be knighted."

Taking a knee in front of Recon, he tapped me once on each shoulder with the hiking pole and then placed a hand on top of my head. "Hence, this day in the lands of Appalachia, thee shall be nam'd Sondance. He who dances with the mountains to honor thee father," he declared solemnly. Handing me the flask, he continued his oration. "Prithee, drinketh the water of life from this sacred vessel. Riseth up and spread ye valorous word over yonder mountains."

I slowly stood amid whistles, applause, and

laughter. "Faire ladies and noble squires, I am humbled by your proclamation. Long may you live and long may you hike," I exclaimed joyfully with a broad smile. Heading back to my tent, I wondered if Recon's dramatic flair was so vividly displayed when he was sober.

At daybreak, or the first light of the traveling lamp, I peered out of tent flaps and watched the gang vanish into the forest. They were starting early to spend more time in Erwin. I marveled at their resiliency. They had partied late into the night, yet managed to rise with the sun. Once upon a time, I could do the same. If only I was forty years younger, I mentally moaned.

I quickly packed up and hit the trail. I had an appointment that afternoon with a reporter from the *Erwin Record*, the local newspaper. On the phone she seemed eager to write an article about Herm's Hike since several family members were suffering from the disease. I looked forward to an easy and hopefully uneventful twelve-mile downhill hike to the front door of Uncle Johnny's hostel.

On the trail, I was still giddy from last night's ceremony. The gang was no longer a group of merry pranksters but my Knights of the Round Table. I couldn't wait to proudly proclaim my new trail name across the land.

Sondance had everything that a hiker could want. It was allegorical, metaphorical, and meteorological. Above all, it was mystical. It represented the "je ne sais quoi" (that attractive, indefinable quality) that reflected the "joie de vivre" (joy of life) personified by the humble hiker previously known as Just Paul. An added bonus was the connotation with the movie *Butch Cassidy and the Sundance Kid.* I savored the "dance" connotation. Ostensibly our lives are simply a great dance on the stage of our design. We choreograph the movements; we select the costumes; we choose the music; and we choose our partners.

Every religion since the dawn of man has used dance in some form to worship a deity. The Hindus call our primal rhythmic energy the sacred dance of our lives. For them, Nataraja (the Lord of Dance) is a depiction of the Shiva (the Supreme Being) as an ecstatic dancer. His dance, the Tandavam, symbolizes the cosmic cycle of creation and destruction, birth and death. I saw all of that in my trail name. Just as every moment of our lives was part of that dance so was every step I took on the AT. "Dance on, Sondance," I shouted joyously to the trees as I journeyed down the path of life.

Thinking about Hindus had me thinking about George Harrison, the quiet Beatle. He found the answers to the mysteries of life in Hare Krishna, the mystical sect of Hinduism. "All religions are branches of one big tree. It doesn't matter what you call Him as long as you call," he once commented. Seconds later, I was singing "My Sweet Lord" with George. I pictured Buddha, Christ, Krishna, Moses, and Muhammad dancing around a campfire in front of a shelter. Afterward, they would have some great stories to share with their trail disciples.

About a mile from the hostel, I heard a wounded cry. Racing up the trail, I found a young woman sitting in the trail with her head in her hands. Tears were dripping from her chin. Behind her was a young man trying to lift her. Hearing my footsteps, he turned in my direction. "Can you help us, mister? She needs to get into town as soon as possible," he implored desperately.

"Yeah, no problem. What can I do for you?" I responded cautiously, not knowing the problem.

"It's her feet. Blisters so bad she can't take a step," he said worriedly.

Sarah and Matt had met at the hiker festival in Hot Springs and started a budding romance, a common love story on the trail. Leaving town, Sarah had a new love to snuggle and new hiking boots that were snug. Instead of turning back at the first blister and risk losing her man, she continued to hike. The boots were now welded to her swollen feet. All I had to offer was some ibuprofen, acetaminophen, and a small first aid kit. What she needed was a medevac to a hospital.

With no cell service, there weren't a lot of options. One of us could stay with Sarah while the other went for help, but a rescue could take hours. Our other choice was to carry Sarah out of the woods. After Matt ditched their backpacks in the brush, we stood Sarah upright and placed her arms over our shoulders.

Progress was agonizingly slow with frequent rest breaks. Every step for Sarah was torture, even though her feet were barely touching the ground. When the pain became unbearable, we changed tactics and used Matt's hiking poles as a makeshift seat. Two things were in our favor: Sarah was a petite woman and we were moving downhill.

We finally arrived at the hostel around 3 o'clock. Already an hour late for my appointment, I called the newspaper. The reporter had left for the weekend but was willing to interview me on Monday. I had to decide if it was worth the wait.

While sitting on the front porch and fretting about my missed opportunity, a car stopped and honked its horn. Matt was behind the wheel with Sarah in the backseat.

"Mind if I ask you for one more favor, Sondance," he said sheepishly. "Would you go with us to the hospital. I might need some help getting Sarah out of the car."

Without hesitating at the sound of my new trail name, I jumped into the passenger seat. Fifteen minutes later, we carried Sarah into the emergency room. About an hour later, we found her resting comfortably on a gurney with her feet propped up. They looked like chunks of raw meat.

Sarah was going to remain over the weekend to monitor any infections. A full recovery could take a month or longer. While she had survived stoically, her hiking boots didn't. Sliced down the ankle and around the sole, they were tossed on a chair with a bloody pair of socks. Love conquers all, but not bad decisions on the trail. New hiking boots were like a new love. They needed to be gradually broken in before a long journey.

Sarah gently clenched my hand and thanked me with tears in her eyes. "Dinner and drinks on me, my friend," Matt said sincerely, shaking my hand. "I couldn't have saved her without you."

Back at the hostel, I secured the last cabin for the night. Trail karma was working its magic. After three nights of sleeping on the cold, hard ground, the lumpy mattress felt like a featherbed. Two months later, I accidentally met up with the couple at a roadside picnic area in Pennsylvania where they were having lunch. Good to their word, dinner (fried chicken) and drinks (cold beer) were on them. While Matt had continued to hike, Sarah was off the trail, continuing to heal. They hoped to reunite in Maine. On the trail, good karma usually resulted in a good meal.

Chapter 9

Homes away from Home

(Erwin to Abby's Place)

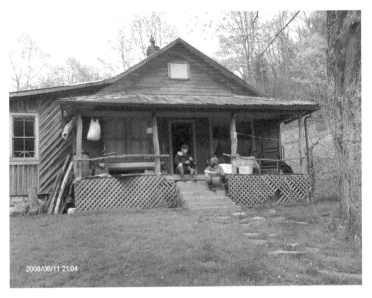

The rustic Greasy Creek Friendly, an answer to prayers in many ways.

That night Uncle Johnny's was overflowing with hikers. From the festive atmosphere, it was obvious most hikers were planning to party throughout the weekend. For me, one night of celebration was enough. The following morning, glad to be alone, I headed for the trail armed with a new camera. Over the next eighty-three miles, there were five hostels, all part of the great "hostel run." I didn't want to straggle and miss out like I did at Elmer's.

Crossing the Nolichucky River, my thoughts drifted back to the past week. The infinite power of love had been dramatically displayed. Pure and true love could move mountains. It was an invisible, immeasurable, and boundless force that connected us to the universe. Jenna, Mist-on-the-Mountain, Hog Greer, and Sarah and Matt had found love accepted, rejected, projected, and subjected in some combination. Before disappearing under the forest canopy, I thought about the tragic fate of the beloved Mary and shuddered. It was a shameful love story that bordered on unimaginable madness.

On September 13, 1916, Mary, the five-ton African elephant and star of the Sparks Brothers Circus, was hanged to death from a derrick crane in the railyard at Erwin. To the delight of over 2,000 townspeople, she thrashed the air with bloodcurdling shrieks until she fell silent. The previous day while parading to a watering hole, she trampled an assistant to death after stopping for a piece of watermelon. Red Eldridge, drifter and apprentice trainer, had unintentionally prodded an abscessed tooth.

Stopping to rest at the Beauty Spot, I sat down and leaned against my backpack. When I tried to stand, I couldn't move. From the waist down, I was paralyzed. No sharp pain, only a dull ache in my right hip and lower back. Thinking it was just a muscle cramp, I decided to rest a little longer. Too embarrassed to ask for help, I simply nodded and waved to passing hikers. Ten minutes later, I still couldn't move. Panic, not pain, was setting in.

Reaching into my backpack, I took two ibuprofens and waited. Nothing happened! Fifteen minutes later, two more pills. Still nothing! Fifteen minutes later, two more pills. Not wanting to overdose, I leaned back and waited nervously for the medication to be absorbed into my bloodstream. While rummaging through my pack, I also discovered another love note from Brite. I was instantly feeling better. The small yellow piece of paper that whispered words of love was my only connection with my real world back in Maryland. I would read it over and over until the next mail drop when Brite would surreptitiously stash another note among the contents. It was my own love story, one as powerful as any found on the trail. It always gave me the strength to keep moving forward.

Gradually, the ache subsided, and I was finally able to stand. Other than being stiff from the cold ground, I showed no ill effects from the trauma or the medication. I comfortably hiked another mile and a half to a campsite. With a severe storm due later in the afternoon, hikers were feverishly pitching their tents. While I searched for a suitable spot, a young solo hiker arrived on the scene.

"Anyone heading to the Greasy?" he asked excitedly.

"I'm game," I answered after finding the best tent sites taken. "Do you think we can make it before the storm hits?"

"No problem at all. I've been there before. If the weather gets bad I know a shortcut," he boasted.

My new hiking partner was Superman, a recent college graduate in his early twenties who was headed to the Harbour Mountain hostel to meet his father for a section hike. A former collegiate hockey player, he was a strong hiker who moved briskly. From the start, I was chasing his footsteps and falling behind.

"Yeah, no problem usually becomes the biggest problem out here," I mumbled angrily under my breath, now leery about putting my fate in the hands of a trail baby. To ease my troubled mind, probably his also, Superman decided music would be the perfect antidote. From his backpack, he retrieved two small speakers and attached them to the back of the pack. The playlist from his I-pod was an enjoyable mix of pop, rock, jazz, and folk that I recognized. For the time being, I was singing joyfully, walking not worrying. If nothing else, Superman had good tastes in music.

About an hour later, my superhero suddenly stopped dead in his tracks and turned off the music. "I think we're lost. I haven't seen a white blaze in a while," he said tersely. As he checked his map, dark clouds gathered overhead.

Seeing the worried look on my face, he insisted that we were not lost, just off the trail. "All we have to do is backtrack a little, pick up this trail and we'll be back on the AT in minutes," he said, running his finger along the map. I had no choice but to follow, keep the pace, and trust in my guide. Being lost in the wilderness with someone was better than being lost in the wilderness alone. Fifteen minutes later, my faith was rewarded. We were once again following white blazes. Superman had come to the rescue.

We eventually reached an abandoned road that led to the Greasy Creek Friendly Hostel. As a cold, hard rain began to fall, I knocked on the back door of the weathered, ramshackle country house.

Seconds later, Cee Cee, proprietor of the hostel, welcomed us with a warm smile. Stepping inside, we were instructed that house rules first required a shower. Not a bad policy since I smelled liked wet dog. With an overflowing crowd, Superman and I were lucky to find space in the drafty but dry bunkhouse.

The hostel was named for the nearby mineral-laden creek that left the skin feeling slimy or slippery. Cee Cee added the "friendly" tag in response to her maniacal neighbor who lived across the dirt road. For unknown reasons, he was vehemently resolved to shut down the hostel at any cost. Through the late evening and early morning hours, he blasted country music from outdoor speakers, raced his motorcycle along the road, yelled and screamed incoherently, and shined lights on the property. It was a Hatfield-McCoy feud that law enforcement largely ignored, resulting in a volatile situation that could explode in violence at any time. To light the fuse, there were a number of "tough guy" hikers, easily pissed off, who simply wouldn't put up with the neighbor's nonsense.

Like any hostel, the house rules reflected the idiosyncrasies of the owner. Greasy Creek was no different. Small signs were posted throughout the house about the do's and don'ts. Price lists for food and services were posted in plain view. Cee Cee kept a running tab for each hiker that included tax at checkout time. Being holed up in a mountain outpost miles from a convenience store, I couldn't complain.

With the storm stalling over the mountains, everyone extended their stay. On my second day, I firmly planted myself on a couch with the other guests and watched trucking comedies such as *Smokey and the Bandit* and *Convoy*. Hikers hooted and howled for hours. Burt Reynolds was a rousing hit with the millennials. For dinner, I made the exhausting road trip to Johnson City for the all-you-can-eat Chinese buffet that included a pocketful of fortune cookies for the trail.

That evening while sitting on the front porch with spectacular views of Roan Mountain, I had a chance to talk with Cee Cee, a fellow baby boomer. Recently divorced, she was running the hostel by herself, desperately hoping to generate enough revenue to repair the infrastructure. To her, the hostel was a labor of love. Like other hostel owners, she loved the trail and those who hiked it.

As a recent convert to Messianic Judaism, we talked about searching for spirituality beyond the rigid precepts of mainstream religion. After telling her my guardian angel story, she reached out and gently placed her hand on top of mine. "If it wasn't a guardian angel, it was definitely a messenger from God," she confided. "Guardian angels can certainly be an answer to a prayer, but always remember, you could be the answer to someone else's prayer."

That night in the bunkhouse, those words lingered in my mind like sacred incense. "Let me be the answer to someone's prayer," I whispered faintly. I breathed those words until they seeped into my soul. They transcended religion and reflected the compassion that is the core of every spiritual journey. Closer to my religious upbringing, they manifested the Prayer of Saint Francis, which was my father's favorite. That was one creed that should be part of everyone's "code of the road" as they journey along life.

The following day, I hiked from Roan Mountain back to the hostel with a young, portly, grinning, bearded hiker named Slackpack. His goal was to slackpack as much of the AT as possible. Having to hitchhike to and from trailheads, he claimed that his secret weapon for a ride was his irresistible, friendly face that should be hosting a children's TV show. While standing on a deserted country road in the rain, I had my doubts, but Slackpack was as good as advertised. The first car that we saw stopped to give us a ride.

At the top of the mountain, we walked over to the former site of the Cloudland Hotel for a quick history lesson. Built in 1885, the legendary hotel was named for the perpetual clouds that shrouded the mountain. Straddling the North Carolina-Tennessee border, the dining room was reportedly divided into legal and illegal alcohol sections with a white line. Abandoned in 1910, the structure eventually succumbed to the harsh weather and crumpled to the ground.

"It would have made a great hostel," I joked.

"At least it would have been easier to get a shot and a beer," Slackpack cackled in reply. Our hostel was located in a dry county.

Our ten-mile downhill footrace with daypacks took around four hours. Back at the hostel, Slackpack immediately bonded with the three new arrivals. Early yesterday evening, they had left the trail, hoping to hitch a ride to the hostel. With rain and darkness falling and hopelessly lost, they sought shelter inside abandoned automobiles at a junkyard. "Cold, dry, and somewhat comfortable, depending on your choice of make and model," one of the hikers hilariously remarked. I looked at Slackpack and smiled. He had the road face they sorely needed.

Despite the good times at the hostel, there was

revolution in the air. While Cee Cee was running errands, some of the hikers openly whined about the house rules and prices. "Nickeled and dimed to death," they grumbled. I bit my tongue, hoping to avoid the debate, because I had heard the same remarks at Uncle Johnny's.

"What do you think about this place, Sondance?" one of the hikers finally asked as if I was the wise elder.

"All the hostels have their own quirks. You need to embrace them as a unique part of the trail," I replied calmly but sternly. "This place is just a simple wayside refuge for the weary traveler. Cee Cee just wants to meet expenses and make enough to live on. You're not going to find a more caring person on the trail." My remarks were met with silence.

The next morning I paid my bill for three nights, two shuttle rides, and a wheelbarrow full of snacks. I noticed that nobody else was leaving. Maybe my scolding did some good. Outside Cee Cee started up the rusted four-wheel-drive vehicle with a screwdriver, and we headed to the top of Roan Mountain.

"Hey, I think I see your angel up ahead waiting for you." She chuckled with her trademark bear hug as we departed. "See you in Damascus."

On the trail in a swirling mist, I didn't see any angels or any hikers. My thoughts remained with Cee Cee and her plight to save the hostel. I hoped she was successful. Hostel owner, poet, and writer, she was a beautiful soul. I wondered how anyone could complain about a hostel that had its own theme song:

Have a smiley face day at the Greasy Creek Friendly,
Have a butterfly day at the Greasy Creek Friendly,

Dreams can come true at the Greasy Creek Friendly,
Have a super butterfly day!

Beyond Roan Mountain, the Roan Highlands stretched for another five miles. "Bald and blind, but the mountain doesn't mind. Wind and rain, and I'm going insane," I blabbered merrily as sweat and rain stung my eyes. I was amazed at how witty I could be in such dire situations. Again, my breathable, waterproof jacket could not breathe fast enough to keep pace with my legs.

I stopped at Overmountain Shelter for a lunch break. The large barn, which could house twenty hikers or more, had been the backdrop for the 1989 movie *Winter People*, a love story about two feuding families in a small mountain town during the Great Depression. Thinking about Cee Cee and her neighbor, I concluded that feuding should be recognized as the official sport of Appalachia.

Inside I startled a hiker who was on his knees intensely studying a map. I had finally come face to face with the AT phantom. Sushi, as the Japanese hiker had been playfully named, roamed the trail like a ghost, randomly appearing at various locations. Since he spoke very little English and avoided hostels, hikers didn't have a clue who he was or where he was going. Today, he didn't have a clue where he was going either. Waving me over to his side, he pointed to the map and shrugged his shoulders with a grunt.

"We're here," I said, grabbing his finger and placing it on the map.

"Ah, good," he replied. Without another word, he quickly folded his map and threw on this backpack. As he hurried out the door, I wondered what my father would have done in my place. I comically pictured him pointing to a spot on the map that would have marched Sushi off a cliff. Although my father never spoke disparagingly about the Japanese, I never knew if he had forgiven them for the war that irrevocably changed his life. With him being a devout Catholic, I believed that he had, but he would never buy a Japanese car. I think that he may have considered that to be un-American.

Hours later, I climbed Hump Mountain, the last bald of the day, completely out of gas. My boots felt like concrete blocks. Stopping to rest, I considered spending the night on the bald, but the hostel was only five miles away. I snapped open one of my fortune cookies that read, "Sometimes travel to new places leads to great transformation." Time to keep hiking.

Wearily trudging along, I repeated the two popular trail mantras for motivation: "Lord, you pick 'em up, and I'll put 'em down," and "No pain, no rain, no Maine." Neither worked. Instead my encounter with Sushi had me again thinking about my father. Right about now, he was probably sitting in the community room, staring blankly at his fellow patients while trying to decipher what was happening around him.

"What are you, some kind of popsicle?" I scolded myself, using my father's word when he blithely chided someone for quitting. "You're pathetic, just pathetic, a whole new flavor," I cried out angrily.

I was walking in a Garden of Eden, surrounded by the beauty of nature, and bellyaching about being tired and wet. Back at the nursing home, there were patients who would gladly sell their souls to trade places with me for an hour. My tirade was an excellent motivator. Now with each step, I pictured my father and his nursing home companions walking behind me.

"Come on, Herm! Come on, Bob! Come on, Paul (the names of my father's first and last roommates)! The bunkhouse is just around the bend," I shouted, waving them on. I comically pictured this group of weary old men merrily shuffling along the trail with beaming smiles, *If only to have them for an hour or a day, I'd crawl to Katahdin,* I thought, echoing the sentiments of Wendy.

At dusk, I staggered into the Mountain Harbour Hostel. Greeting me with a beer as if he was expecting my arrival was Jorel, father of Superman. He said that Superman had opted to stay another day at the hostel to wait out the storm. I had no doubt it was to wait out the party. He seemed to have an affinity for that part of trail life.

Unlike the Greasy Creek Friendly, the Mountain Harbour had a bunkhouse with heat and running water. Booked for the night, Mary, one of the owners with her husband, Terry, told me that I could sleep in the stable beneath the bunkhouse. If it was good enough for Mary and Joseph, then it was good enough for me.

As I was stacking hay bales in the tack room for my bed, Mary found me with good news. I had a real bed for the night. Two hikers with reservations couldn't make it over Hump Mountain in the storm. Quietly, I thanked my imaginary hiking buddies for their inspiration.

The next morning I feasted on a breakfast spread that included French toast with maple syrup, shrimp and grits, egg casserole, potatoes with green beans, biscuits and gravy, kielbasa, poached pears, strawberry cake, monkey bread, fresh coffee, and juice. If there was an award for the best breakfast on the AT, Mary and Terry had my vote. With a full stomach, I was ready to hike.

Late that afternoon under an overcast sky, I came to a park bench, a rather odd sight in the middle of the forest. With wood slats and a metal frame, the bench was more suited for a town square than a trail. Engraved in the slats was the following inscription: "In loving memory, Ron G. Frey 'Vango,' who received so little yet gave so much." Dropping my backpack and grabbing a water bottle, I cheerfully took a seat and enjoyed a delightful view of Hump Mountain in the distance.

Just north of the bench, I spotted the bent tree and followed the power-line trail. As I approached a clearing in the woods, I heard the sound of a circular saw. Abby's Place was under construction. Looking up, I spotted a worker on the second floor. "I'll be down in a few minutes. Just finishing up for the day," shouted Scotty, owner and hostel architect.

"Open for business?" I asked anxiously when he reappeared.

"Not officially, but you can spend the night for free. Come on, I'll give you a tour," he replied cheerfully, obviously delighted to show off his labor of love. The hostel closed last year with the death of Ron Frey, a father-like figure who had been the guiding force in Scotty's life.

Like myself, Scotty was out to prove himself a "good son." He was renovating the structure as a memorial to Ron. Although Ron never hiked the trail, he became the consummate trail angel after his retirement. As expected the memorial bench had its own story. When seated, you could see the steeple of Ron's beloved church on the mountain horizon. After Scotty's explanation about the bench, I added a new commandment to the AT handbook of etiquette: When you come to a park bench in the middle of the woods, sit on it. Sometimes it can connect a dot or two.

"You and I have a virtue in common. We are the good sons," I gushed before telling him about Herm's Hike. Deeply touched by my comments, he thanked me with tears in his eyes.

That night I had the bunkhouse to myself. The finished first floor had two bunk beds, a working computer, a disconnected rotary phone, and a stove, all covered in sawdust. After dinner, I exchanged e-mails with Brite and played a few games on the computer. It passed the time, but what I really wanted was to hear Brite's voice. With no cell service and the wires on the phone disconnected, it was time to improvise.

With some tinkering, I found that by pressing the wires to the inside terminals on the phone, I could get a dial tone. Seconds later, Brite answered the phone. There was nothing more soothing than the voice of my sweetheart. Despite my dreary surroundings and rain beating against the windows, I went to bed with the comforting thought that all was well on the home front. With a loving family, I wouldn't trade places with anyone in the world, but sometimes I envied the younger hikers who had no family obligations. They were vagabond gypsies, moving like clouds along a mountain trail. Unencumbered by the realities of everyday life, they had the freedom of youth. I often daydreamed about how it would have been to hike just out of college. No job, no wife, no kids, just a great adventure to be devoured and savored. I wondered if my father felt that way when he was finally able to enlist in the army and follow his dream. Pondering his enthusiasm for the simplest pleasures in life, I had no doubt that he did.

Chapter 10
A Ghostly Visitation
(Abby's Place to Vandeventer Shelter)

After an enjoyable twelve-mile hike under cloudy skies with no rain, a rare weather event, I found myself standing in front of a rustic two-story cottage. Nestled in the woods, covered in ivy and surrounded by shrubs and plants, the building seemed ideally suited for an Irish pub or a home for retired leprechauns. The penultimate stop on the great hostel run was Kincora. Opened in 1997 by Bob Peoples, a retired air force officer, it had become legendary for its hospitality.

Once inside, I immediately noticed the walls were papered with hundreds of photos from thru-hikers. I could only hope to be among the gallery one day. In the kitchen, a staff member cordially welcomed me to Bob's home. Not surprisingly, Bob, noted for his trail work, was out with a crew. After a pasta lunch, last night's leftovers, I was given a tour of the house and the grounds that included the famous tree house.

Later in the day, I was formally introduced to the white-haired, white-mustached owner with the ever-present baseball cap. With a firm handshake and a twinkle in his eye, the larger-than-life trail leprechaun inquired about my hike. Being a veteran, he quickly found a prominent spot on the kitchen wall for my flyer.

After dinner, a small group of hikers followed Bob and Baltimore Jack to the front porch for story time. Well into the night, two of the greatest trail raconteurs had us laughing about nude, rude, prude, lewd, and stewed hikers.

One arrogant hiker insisted on a free tab because he was the grandson of Earl Shaffer. When Bob pointed out that Earl never had any children, the hiker vehemently claimed that Bob was the charlatan who never knew the real Earl Shaffer. Earl the Younger was literally tossed out the front door like a drunken cowboy in a TV western and told never to come back.

Baltimore Jack, who was helping Bob for a few weeks, took his trail name from the Bruce Springsteen song "Hungry Heart." Sometime in the '80s, Leonard Adam Tarlin, a college graduate with a degree in history, simply walked away from his wife and young daughter and found his calling on the trail. The hard-living, hard-drinking wanderlust, who resembled Jerry Garcia, had thru-hiked nine times. He was trail royalty. In the audience that night was Superman. Several times, I glanced at him to see his reaction to Jack's funnier stories. I wondered if someday he might lay claim to Jack's crown.

In the morning, the effervescent Baltimore Jack prepared blueberry pancakes for breakfast. Before heading out, I opened my last fortune cookie. It said, "Spirit guides accompany you." I could have used that one on Blood Mountain. Nonetheless, it was a good omen.

At the Laurel Fork Falls, I stopped for a photo

break. After a few quick shots, I tucked away my camera and hastily retrieved my Gore-Tex jacket. It was starting to rain. Hurriedly I followed the path along the creek for a couple of miles until it reached a bend.

Walking along a narrow ledge next to the creek, the rain suddenly turned into a blinding deluge. With cold water trickling in at the collar of my jacket, I reached around with my left and yanked hard on the hood string. Instantly, I slipped on the wet rock and tumbled. Falling about six feet in slow motion, I splashed the creek and landed on my back. Looking up at the sky, I felt the cold water rushing over my body. Except for my head, I was submerged. Rolling over and quickly jumping to my feet, I sloshed downriver to retrieve my hiking poles.

After staggering ashore, I slowly gained my composure and did a quick physical examination. There were no apparent cuts or broken bones, only some scrapes on my hands. With trembling hands, I inspected my backpack. Other than being filled with water, there was no damage. My sleeping bag, spare clothes, and some other essentials were in waterproof bags. With a sigh of relief, I realized that my backpack saved my life. If I had landed on my side or face, I could have been knocked unconscious and drowned.

After emptying my boots and changing into dry socks, I decided to push forward to the next hostel instead of turning back. Dazed and frightened from my brush with death, I followed the trail along the creek until I reached the next blaze. Upon close inspection, it appeared the blaze had once been blue and painted white or vice-versa. Either way it did not appear to be true white. Hopefully I was only confused and not lost.

Just as I was ready to pull out my map, I noticed a woman standing on the trail about twenty yards away. She stood quietly, smoking a cigarette while staring into the woods. Tall and skinny with stringy blonde hair, she appeared to be in her late teens or early twenties. Wearing jeans, a fleece top, and no hat, she wasn't dressed for the weather. But that didn't matter, I was just glad to find someone on the trail.

"Excuse me, do you think you can help me out? I think I'm lost," I said nervously.

"Where do you want to go?" she asked after a long pause, still staring straight ahead.

"I fell into the creek and need to get back on the trail," I replied. "Oh, by the way, my name is Paul," I added, hoping to ease the tension.

"Well, you're already on a trail, and my name is Regina," she replied tersely, still standing like a statue.

An ice-cold shiver ran down my spine, raising the hair on the back of my neck. I had an aunt on my mother's side whose religious name had been Sister Regina. After taking her final vows, the young nun was assigned as a missionary to a colored parish in Alabama. Two years later in 1944, she contracted tuberculosis. At Johns Hopkins Hospital, the doctors told my grandparents that if they had seen her six months earlier, they could have saved her life. A few weeks later, Sister Regina was dead at the age of twenty-four. She was buried next to the founder of the order, Mother Colette Hilbert, an honor whose explanation was lost in time.

Trying to collect my thoughts, I wasn't sure what to do or say next. I was scared after falling into the creek; now I was spooked.

"Am I dead?" I blurted. For the first time since I fell into the creek, the sobering thought that I might actually be dead crossed my mind. Maybe I was knocked unconscious and drowned. Perhaps, this woman was my spirit messenger to carry me across to the other side.

"Are you dead what?" she quipped still staring straight ahead.

"A, a, a, dead like dead lost," I stammered, scrambling for words that didn't make me sound like a lunatic.

"Hardly. Just follow my directions and you'll be back on the trail in no time," she scoffed.

"Hardly dead or hardly lost, or somewhere in between isn't a good place to be on a day like today," I mumbled to myself.

Following her instructions, I slipped along a steep muddy trail, falling several times. About a half an hour later, now covered in mud, I rounded a corner to a familiar sight. Just ahead was Regina, still staring and still smoking. I had hiked in a circle. Once again, I approached her and asked for directions. This time she offered an alternate route, a blue-blazed trail that led to a parking lot and the main road into Hampton.

"Do you mind if I ask you what you're doing out here?" I inquired curiously, part of me still not convinced I wasn't dead. This time I stood a little closer, hoping to glimpse some slight detail that might solve the origin of this mystery woman. Leaning slightly forward, I spotted an insignia on her fleece jacket. It was too small to read, but it appeared similar to the crown on a Crown Royal whiskey bottle.

"Looks like I was waiting for you," she deadpanned

without a glance.

If she hadn't been standing in the middle of a forest, I would have assumed that she was blind. I again thanked her and followed the trail. Turning around for one last look, she was still standing in the rain with a cigarette in hand, no doubt waiting for the next lost soul. Farther down the trail, I came to a parking lot just as the heavens opened up with a wall of water. The lot was empty. I stood there dumbfounded. *Who was that woman and where did she come from?* I wondered.

"Get in before you drown," shouted the driver of a pickup truck that skidded to a stop next to me.

"I think I already have," I replied morosely as rivulets of rain ran down the sleeves of my jacket.

A few miles down the road, the driver deposited me at the doorstep of the Braemar Castle Hostel, named after the famous castle in Scotland. With hardwood floors, painted walls, private rooms, and a large living area with a full kitchen, the place was more of a hotel than a hostel. It was bright, airy, clean, and empty. There wasn't a hiker to be found. With numerous empty rooms, there was an eerie, haunting feeling in the air. I felt as if I was standing in the fictional Overlook Hotel, the setting for the horror-suspense movie *The Shining*. Any second, I expected to see Jack Nicholson careening around the corner with an axe in his hand.

After my near-death experience, I needed to be around people. More than that, I needed to be back on the trail and moving forward. I quickly laundered my hiking clothes and scrubbed my backpack. Under a threatening sky, I hitched a ride to the trailhead.

The hike through the watershed at Watauga Dam

included a number of paved roads, scenic overlooks, and a walk across the dam. At the time it was opened in 1948, the man-made mountain was one of the largest earth dams in the country, measuring 318 feet in height and 900 feet in length. At a small parking lot, I stopped to eat an early dinner when a pickup truck with a "Proud to be Cherokee" bumper sticker pulled in.

Out stepped two young men sporting high-top moccasins with hunting knives strapped to the outside. With bronze-colored skin, high cheekbones, and silky black ponytails, it wasn't difficult to identify them as descendants of the Cherokee Nation.

Being the only people in the lot, we chatted as they unloaded their bloodhounds for a run in the woods. They were anxiously waiting graduation from high school in a couple of months and planning to study computer science at the local community college in the fall. Just two young men excited to begin the next phase of their lives. I had the same feeling fifty-years ago. I liked the pair even more when they quickly associated my trail name with Butch Cassidy. Like me, they were big movie fans. They loved westerns as long as they didn't stereotype the Native American as the "noble savage." And like me, *Dances with Wolves* was one of their favorite flicks. As I left, I wished them success in their careers. Thinking back, I realized my wish from Blood Mountain had come true. I had met the heirs to the Trail of Tears. I knew their ancestors had to be proud.

At dusk, I arrived at Vandeventer Shelter and claimed the last space. Wearily unrolling my sleep pad and bag, I changed into my sleeping clothes and zipped up for the evening. During the bedtime story hour in the darkness of the shelter, I recounted my "man overboard" story to the amazement of my bunkmates.

"It's no coincidence that your backpack is an Osprey," a female voice rang out. "The osprey is your spirit guide on your spiritual journey." I wasn't convinced about my spirit animal from a self-proclaimed New Age mystic who read tarot cards and palms, but I was certain my Osprey was a lifesaver. It could be marketed as a backpack and personal flotation device. Just as I dozed off, a furious storm hit the area with pulsating waves of rain that created a symphony of percussion. Warm and dry in my bed of feathers, I paid little attention to the raging tempest outside.

About an hour later, I was rousted from my sleep with the arrival of three hikers who got caught in the storm. They politely asked if there was any space, and hikers graciously complied by squeezing closer. Every inch of the floor was now covered with a sleeping bag. A little after midnight, I was jolted from my sleep by the sounds of heavy thunder directly overhead. The cannonade was literally rattling the rafters. Lightning cracked the sky and speared the earth, exploding in flashes of blinding light. *Albert Mountain*, I thought in horror.

The rain pounded relentlessly on the tin roof like a long roll on a snare drum. One by one, hikers rolled over on their stomachs to peer into the darkness. Every few seconds, I checked to make sure that my body was not off the rubber sleeping pad and touching the wood floor. It might be my only chance to survive a lightning strike. Surrounded by the cacophony of nature's unbridled wildness, we held a collective breath and waited for the storm to pass. When the forest fell silent, we rolled back over and exhaled a collective sigh of relief.

I closed my eyes but couldn't sleep. My mind raced with questions of doubt. The darkest day on the trail had become the darkest night of the soul. Reflecting on the day's events, I realized that I was lucky to be alive. Today may have been nature's way of telling me to go home. Hundreds of miles away, my father was slowly dying and my wife was alone. I didn't need any other reasons to leave the trail behind.

Who was I kidding with this noble cause? Maybe I was needed more at home than on the trail. And these people that I was meeting on the trail in my hour of need, were they real people, real angels, or real hallucinations? Was the stress of hiking alone causing me to lose my mind? Long-distance hikers have cracked under the mental and physical stress. Was my name going to be the next one on the list?

I had no answers. Perhaps, this day was another spiritual revelation on the road to that mystical transformation. Time would tell, but I didn't know how many more days like today I could endure. But one thing was certain. If these apparitions were angels, they weren't dressed for the occasion. They needed to expand their spiritual wardrobe to fit the occasion. I chuckled at that thought of angels being categorized, classified, or deputized by religious scholars. Those who claimed to have angelic insight obviously had never met a real one. Forget all that nonsense about the nine choirs of angels. An angel is an angel. I had stumbled upon two. I didn't need to see their IDs or union cards.

At first light, I blearily crawled out of the shelter like a shell-shocked soldier after an apocalyptic battle and inspected the carnage. In the morning stillness, the only sound was water dripping from the trees. A faint odor of burning wood hung in the humid air. I was amazed that the shelter hadn't floated away. If I had a cigarette, I would have smoked it like a weary combat veteran in a war movie. Yet, despite the bleak surroundings, I was ecstatic. I was going on furlough. Damascus was only two days away, a day and a half if I hustled.

Chapter 11
A Field of Dreams
(Vandeventer Shelter to Damascus, VA)

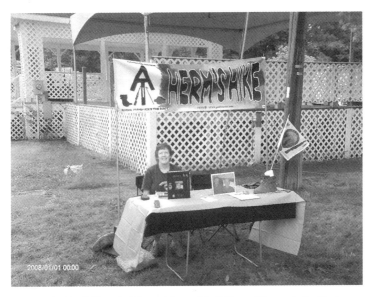

Brite behind Herm's Hike tablet at Trail Days. The artistic display attracted attention and donations.

Descending the mountain ridge to Virginia, spring was in full bloom. Patches of white wildflowers carpeted the forest floor like snow. Choirs of songbirds fluttered from the dense brush and filled the air with joyous melodies that were conspicuously absent in the higher elevations.

Under sunny skies, I merrily walked under the sign that welcomed me to Damascus, home of Trail Days and the mecca for past, present, and future AT hikers from every corner of the earth.

With three days until the main events on Saturday, the town was already starting to fill. An eccentric mix of Mardi Gras and Woodstock 1969, the festival offered an array of live entertainment (music on almost every corner), free food (just follow the swarm of hikers), free movies (about hiking, of course), free lectures by hiking experts, gear demonstrations, and book signings by trail legends. On the outskirts of town, Tent City provided a nonstop party. By Saturday, the bucolic town of approximately 1,000 residents would be bursting at the seams with nearly 20,000 hikers, vendors, and tourists.

I spent my first night at The Place, a donation hostel operated by the United Methodist Church. The next morning as I was stuffing my sleeping bag into its sack, my overhead bunkie was busily collecting his gear and singing to himself.

"Sometimes, I feel like a motherless child, a long, long way from my home," he crooned softly as I joined along.

"Richie Havens at Woodstock," I blurted out after we had finished.

"Exactly," he gushed.

"I didn't know Richie was Jewish," I joked. The black folksinger had opened the Woodstock Music and Arts Festival on August 15, 1969. His improvised, emotionally charged version of "Freedom" from the spiritual "Motherless Child" became an anthem for the Woodstock generation.

"Everybody who sings and dances to the music of their soul is a Jew at heart," he laughed as he pounded his left chest with his right hand.

"How about soul music like James Brown and the Temptations?" I cackled.

"Yesh, especially Sammy Davis Jr.," he howled. We both laughed at his joke about a famous entertainer who had converted to Judaism.

Itay, trail name No Thai, was a twenty-five-year-old hiker from Israel who had recently finished his mandatory service in the Israeli army. He was in the States on a six-month visa before returning home. We chatted for a few minutes about Woodstock and the AT. My singing partner knew more about American pop culture than most of his American counterparts. Not too many people knew that Sweetwater was the first band to play at Woodstock or that they opened their set with their own version of "Motherless Child."

"You were there in 1969?" Itay stammered excitedly after I ruminated on the heartbreaking fate of the band following the festival. Four months after their performance, their lead singer Nancy Nevins suffered debilitating injuries and damaged vocal chords in an automobile accident.

"Yes and no," I quipped comically. "I'll let you decide after I tell the story."

Itay sat on the edge of his bed and cocked his head to the side with a widening grin.

"But before I begin, remember this was the era before the Internet and cell phones. I was seventeen years old and just out of high school when I heard the rumors about the concert.

"I had arrived in Bethel, New York, site of the festival, unknowingly a week ahead of time. I had quit my summer job and told my parents that I was heading to Ocean City, Maryland, for the weekend with three of my coworkers. When we arrived at Yasgur's farm, workers were frantically trying to finish construction of the stage and staging area. Time was running out. Since I could swing a hammer and saw a board, I was offered a job as a carpenter's helper with no pay. However, if I stayed for the week, I would be fed, housed, and given a backstage pass to the concert. The offer was tempting, but it was impossible for me to stay. The weekend of the festival was my college orientation. Not knowing the fate of the festival, my friends and I camped out for two nights, hung around the area, and then went home.

"Sababa! An awesome story, man. You're just like Joni (Mitchell). You weren't there in body, but you were there in spirit. As a matter of fact, you still are," Itay shrieked gleefully.

I thanked Itay for his inspiriting comment, shouldered my backpack, and headed out the door. Itay was busy gathering his belongings and singing "Motherless Child" with renewed gusto.

After updating my trail journal on the hiker computer at the town library, I stopped next door at Trails Consignment to kill time. As I browsed the merchandise, the owner, Vicki, entered from the back. "Just out of the military?" she asked in response to my short hair.

"Once upon a time, I did some undergraduate work at USMC, Camp Pendleton campus," I replied.

"Semper Fi," Vicki exclaimed gleefully, reaching out to shake my hand. She was impatiently counting the days until her daughter graduated from boot camp at Parris Island. She was rightfully a proud Marine Corps mom and delighted to meet a fellow marine from the trail.

Before leaving, a treasure caught my eye. A Rawlings catcher's mitt for $10 beckoned with a whisper in my head, "If you buy it, he will come." In a rush of nostalgic fever, I bought it, not questioning the voice about who would come, much less where, when, or why he would come. Being an old catcher, I knew this was a top-of-the-line model that had cost around $100 when new. In high school, I had owned a similar glove.

"I've seen some strange hiking gear. I'm just wondering how you're going to use a catcher's mitt on the Appalachian Trail," Vicki said with a bemused smile.

"Maybe a pillow or pot holder. I'm not sure myself. All I know is that I have to have it," I replied whimsically.

Grabbing my mitt, I walked a few blocks to Backer Park, a small cinder-block ballpark with a low-slung grandstand behind home plate. To my disappointment, the field was empty. There would be no ball game today, not even a catch. I took a seat in the stands and gazed at the grass. Pounding the pocket of my glove with my fist, I wondered how many big league dreams had lived and died at this humble ball field.

I closed my eyes and waited for the answer. Ever so slowly, the blurred images of a once-promising high school baseball career came into focus. The memory washed over my body like sacred water from the river of life. I reached out and touched it with the hands of a young teenager who just wanted to play ball.

During my junior year, my varsity career as the starting catcher ended after one game. On opening day, I went 1 for 3 with a double, an RBI, and a stolen base in a win. In the second game, I was benched after four innings in favor of the senior back-up catcher. I never played another inning that season. During my senior year, I was benched in favor of the football coach's son.

"This is the hardest decision I had to make in my coaching career," the coach declared when announcing the starting catcher that year. Before the name left his lips, I knew my high school baseball career was over. For the entire season, I dutifully warmed up pitchers and caught batting practice. Instead of playing baseball, I looked forward to drinking beer like a major leaguer on the weekends with the guys from my neighborhood. I needed something more than aspirin to ease my pain. Emotionally, I was still recovering from being stood-up for the junior prom. High school was not the best of times for me.

To my insouciance, I started the last game of the year. The coach didn't want to risk an injury to the starting catcher in the upcoming championship game. As baseball cannon fodder, I played like it was my last game on earth, getting two hits (an amazing feat for someone who never faced live pitching during the season), driving in three runs, and stealing two bases. I could only imagine what might have been.

Faint cheers and jeers broke the astral spell. Frisbee players were taking the field for a game of Frisbee baseball. Today Backer Park would not be my "field of dreams." The sacred waters had receded, leaving a tidal pool of bittersweet memories. I walked back to the hostel with my mitt feeling like it was made of stone.

After a tiring day of pounding the streets to

promote Herm's Hike, I returned to the hostel, grabbed my backpack, and waited on the front porch of the Hikers Inn for my next hiking partner. Doc, a physician's assistant in the Coast Guard, planned to spend the night and take a day hike. What thru-hiker could say no to a personal physician, if for only a day?

Brite and I had first met Doc in 2007 when we sailed aboard the Coast Cutter *Healy* on a dependents cruise. The soft-spoken, mild-mannered officer with an engaging sense of humor welcomed us with open arms as an intimate member of the *Healy* family. He had nothing but praise for our daughter Cynthia, one of his shipmates.

The next morning we shuttled about six miles out of town and hiked back on the AT. Before beginning, I bestowed him with the trail name of Holliday as in Doc Holliday, the famous gambler, gunfighter, and dentist. Doc loved it, especially the connotation with the Old West. As we walked and talked, I detected nervousness in his voice.

"So I guess you want to hear about the *Healy*?" he finally asked in a hesitating tone.

"Ready if you are," I assured. I had always wanted to hear his account of the tragedy but respected his privacy. When the time was right, he would tell his story. Today in the woods, surrounded by the serenity of the nature, the time had arrived.

Sailing out of Seattle, the icebreaker *Healy* was the Coast Guard's largest vessel at 420 feet in length. Her primary mission was to support research expeditions to the Arctic Circle for up to six months of the year.

On August 17, 2006, two Coast Guard divers descended into the icy waters through a hole in the ice for a training dive. The ship was 490 miles north of Barrow, Alaska. In accordance with regulations, Doc was on the ice with the dive cadre as the senior officer. It was merely a formality. During the exercise, all diving decisions were the sole responsibility of the senior diver.

Minutes into dive, safety lines attached to the divers peeled wildly through the hands of the dive tenders. In seconds, the divers plunged over two hundred feet as if they were falling off a mountain. Attempting to compensate for cold-water buoyancy issues, they had packed additional weight that could not be jettisoned in an emergency. Both divers had lost consciousness and suffered ruptured lungs.

With the divers back on the ice, Doc immediately began life-saving procedures that continued aboard the ship's medical facility. Despite his heroic efforts, the two divers could not be saved. Physically and emotionally exhausted, Doc did not relish the job of cleaning up the makeshift operating room that looked like a combat field hospital.

At that moment, a newly minted ensign from the Coast Guard Academy named Cynthia Travers appeared in the doorway and asked if she could help. The cleanup job was hers. In the darkest hour of his life, Doc found an angel at his door. For that he would be forever grateful.

"I always felt that I should have done more. Somehow changed the outcome," Doc added wistfully, his voice trailing off.

"Doc, when the skies are clear at night, I slide my head out of the tent and stare at stars, imagining the points of light are events in my life. And those dots, no matter how tragic some may seem, connect to some goodness in the universe, even if we don't see it. But rest assured, one day we will."

Doc just nodded in agreement, probably wondering when did Cindy's dad became a mystic. I was wondering the same thing. For the rest of the hike, we bantered back and forth with sea stories and trail tales. That evening at dinner, Doc's mood seemed much brighter. The trail had worked its magic. The mountain had healed an aching heart.

After Doc departed the following morning, I visited the Mountain Laurel Inn where Brite and I would be staying that weekend. With breakfast being served, Leslie, the gracious owner, asked me if I wanted to eat. What hiker who had already lost nearly fifteen pounds wouldn't want fresh eggs, bacon, and orange juice?

Two couples sitting nearby asked me about my hike. When I told them about Herm's Hike, one of the ladies asked me my trail name. "Sondance, he who dances with the mountains in honor of the father," I replied proudly.

"Do you mean heavenly father or earthly father?" the woman asked politely.

"Both," I responded, quickly grasping the double meaning of my trail name.

At that point, Judy asked if she could pray with me. I graciously agreed. With the other couple, we joined hands in a prayer circle as Judy beseeched God to lead and safeguard me on the trail. I was left teary eyed.

A few minutes later, Judy returned to my table.

"Do you mind if I ask you a personal question?"

"Not at all," I replied casually, wondering what was on her mind.

"Have you ever thought about getting Alzheimer's since your father has the disease?" she asked candidly.

"The thought has crossed my mind a few times since I've been on the trail. It's been just one of a million thoughts, though," I replied guardedly, not knowing where the conversation was going.

"Do you mind if I pray with you again?" she asked gently. Thinking that prayers are like money in the bank for withdrawal in an emergency, I readily agreed.

Gently placing one hand on my forehead and the other on my shoulder, Judy called out passionately. "Dear Heavenly Father, you sent your only son Jesus Christ to die a horrific death on the cross to atone for our sins and give us eternal life. By the blood of his cross, may you wipe the curse of this dreaded disease from Paul and his family for all eternity. This we pray in your name."

This time tears flowed down my cheeks. Her words had touched my soul. I had never heard a more emotional prayer in my life, and I had heard thousands as an altar boy.

Judy left the room and returned a few minutes later with a check for $100. I humbly thanked her, still teary eyed. "Paul, national publicity will come to you and Herm's Hike. God will see to that, and I feel it through him here today. And at that time, the Holy Spirit will descend upon your tongue and give you the words of the Lord to give to the nation," she confided as if she had just gotten off the phone with God.

Feeling energized by the prayer breakfast, that afternoon I grabbed my mitt and headed back to the ballpark. This time I found some ballplayers. A man was pitching batting practice to a young boy who appeared to be no more than ten years old. "Eye on the ball. Level swing," the man shouted with each pitch. With only three baseballs, the drill was quickly becoming a game of pitch and fetch.

"Mind if I shag some balls?" I hollered from the grandstand.

"Mister, right about now, I could use all of the help I can get," the man sighed.

After about fifteen minutes of fielding balls, the man turned in my direction. "Your turn to hit if you want. You earned it."

I ran in and picked a bat. After whiffing at the first couple of pitches, I found my stroke and began hitting frozen ropes (line drives) that echoed around the park like rifle shots. Seeing that I was quickly tiring out my fielders, I stopped and asked them if they wanted to play catch. "You go ahead. I'll just watch," replied the father, wiping the sweat from his brow.

The boy and I began with soft tosses at close range. As I gradually stepped back, his throws were now popping leather to his amazement. I never forgot how to catch the ball for that sweet sound.

"Do you play baseball?" the boy asked shyly.

"Played a long time ago. I was a catcher like my dad," I replied. "What about you?"

"I start Little League this year and want to be a catcher. My dad says that's the quickest way to the big leagues. A team never has too many good catchers," he replied, echoing my father's words from fifty years ago.

"Okay, let me see what you got. Get down in your stance and I'll throw you a few pitches." The boy immediately dropped to a catcher's crouch behind home plate and held out his glove as a target. After an imaginary inning with three up and three down, I walked up to him.

"You've got good form and a good arm," I said smiling. "But the one thing you don't have is a catcher's mitt. Here, take mine. You'll grow into it." The boy looked at me in bewilderment and then turned to his father. With a smile breaking across his face, the man nodded his head in approval.

"Thanks, mister. I never had a real catcher's mitt," he replied, caressing the mitt and running his fingers along the smooth leather. I smiled and shook hands with the glove's and the dream's new owner.

My childhood dream of being a baseball player had never really died. Today it was passed along to another young boy with the same aspiration. Baseball karma filled the air like the smell of hot dogs and freshly mowed grass. Today Backer Park had worked its magic as a "Field of Dreams."

Walking back to town, I thought about returning to the ballpark so father and son could hear the rest of my story. Perhaps a full, public confession was required before the baseball gods could grant me final absolution.

When people asked me why *Field of Dreams* was my favorite movie of all time, I usually told them it was a greatest baseball movie if not the greatest movie ever made and left it at that. I was reluctant to tell the truth and share my secret. Ray Kinsella, the main character in the movie, and I were kindred souls.

Ray and I were officially English majors in the late '60s who in reality majored in the sixties. We both committed baseball's mortal sin. We refused to play catch with our fathers. Ray was fourteen at the time, and I was seventeen. In early spring of my senior year, my father asked me if I wanted to work on my throws to second. Filled with teenage angst, most of it directed at my high school, I said no. We never played catch again.

However, unlike Ray, my anger was never directed at my father. He was my hero and role model. Baseball had been our bond. I was the batboy for his teams before I was old enough to actually play for him. As the years rolled by, I always regretted that day in my life. I would have given anything to have it back. Since the debut of the movie in 1989, my penance has been to cry at the end of the movie when Ray takes the field to play catch with the ghost of his father. Religiously twice a year, I watch the movie and go to baseball confession where I confess only that sin.

Back at the inn, Brite, who was waiting on the front porch of the stately Victorian home, leaped from her chair and ran into my arms. Wiping the tears from our eyes, we quickly got down to serious business, the state of the family report. She was fine, the girls were fine, my father was fading a little, and my mother was coping with stoic courage as always. The hike was raising around $250 weekly in donations, and viewership on my trail journal at my website was increasing.

There was one bit of discomforting news. Two weeks ago, a nursing assistant had physically assaulted my father. The attack left him with a black eye, small cuts, and swelling. To prevent this from happening to my father or any other residents, friends and family urged my mother to hire a lawyer, but she steadfastly refused. Fearing litigation might jeopardize my father's care, she decided to let the nursing home handle the situation.

Subsequently, the employee was fired, and the nursing home was off the hook for a lawsuit.

For the next two nights, Brite and I strolled the streets of Damascus hand in hand like two love-struck teenagers. Early Saturday morning, we set up our table for Herm's Hike in the town park with the help of Red Wolf o'da Smoky's, a 1971 thru-hiker, hiking activist, and trail volunteer. When finished, we stepped back to admire our handiwork. It didn't look just good; it looked professional.

In a stroke of marketing genius, Brite had contacted the art teacher at the local high school to see if they needed a project for community hours. Luckily, the teacher was desperately seeking worthy projects. Within a few months, we had a Herm's Hike vinyl banner, two large magnet signs for the car, and numerous posters, all hand-painted and bearing the Herm's Hike logo.

The logo, an advertising brainchild of Brite and myself, featured the familiar stacked A over T against a backdrop of mountains. On one side, pine trees represented the AT. On the other side, palm trees represented the island of Peleliu where my father was wounded during WWII. Leaning on one side of the T was a hiking pole with a pair of hiking boots. On the opposite side was a rifle with a pair of combat boots.

Throughout the day, we distributed information about Alzheimer's disease and talked about Herm's Hike with festivalgoers. Hikers that we had met during our first two weeks stopped to say hello and make a donation. At the end of the day, we had collected $242 in donations.

One special visitor was Bobby Jon Drinkard, star of the popular TV show *Survivor* for two seasons. Brite was delighted to meet the ruggedly handsome journalist and finally get a chance to ask some insider questions about her favorite show. Two days before, I had met Bobby Jon at the Baptist church where he talked about his personal journey of faith. A true southern gentleman, he graciously accepted my invitation to stop by the table.

After breaking down our display, Brite and I headed to the far end of the town for the Hiker Parade, the festival's main event. At 2 o'clock, I joined a thousand hikers from every class year and marched back to the park under a barrage of water balloons, water guns, and hoses from the thousands of spectators lining the street.

On Sunday morning after a hearty hiker's breakfast, Brite drove me back to the trailhead. The mini-vacation was over. It was time to hike.

"Hey, Sondance, I love ya! Be careful out there!" Brite shouted with tears in her eyes. I quickly disappeared into the woods in search of the next white blaze with the loneliest of thoughts: It would be another month and 570 miles between hugs and kisses. I wiped away my own tears, wishing Brite was still by my side, all the time knowing that she had never left. I couldn't wait to empty my backpack and find the next folded piece of paper.

Despite my head start from Damascus, I couldn't out hike the weather. Entering the Grayson Highlands (Virginia's answer to the Scottish Highlands), another storm front stalled over the region with fog and showers. Searching for the wild ponies, southwest Virginia's answer to the famous Chincoteague ponies on the coast, I heard only muffled whinnies in the distance. But I knew they were out there and I knew where to find them.

Blocking the entrance to Thomas Knob Shelter

was a herd of sixteen ponies, including three mares with foals. To enter, I had to wade through a sea of horseflesh, often tapping the ponies with my hiking pole to move them aside. Sensing no snacks were imminent, the alpha mare turned and walked down the trail. The others followed in single file without so much as a grunt, snort, or whinny. I turned and walked up the trail.

Hiking above the tree line, the heavens unleashed a monsoon. I ran for cover at the only shelter. Stepping inside a rock formation, known as Fat Man Squeeze, I quickly discovered that I was not alone.

"Sondance, what brings you to my humble abode?" a voice in the shadows cheerfully announced. Startled, I stepped closer for a better look.

"Floater, I thought you were staying in Damascus for a few more days. But since misery loves company, I'm glad to see you."

Brite and I had first met the affable and unflappable Floater in Franklin. The former army officer from Louisiana had one of the most hard-earned trail names in AT history, and he was darn proud of it. During his first week on the trail, the novice hiker had not yet mastered the skill of trenching. When the first downpour flooded the inside of his tent, he spent the evening floating on his inflatable sleeping pad, an AT waterbed.

Once the rain slackened, I took my leave. Floater opted to wait and stay dry. Who could blame him?

Chapter 12
Walkin' Off the War
(Damascus to Daleville, VA)

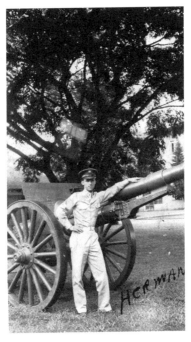

PFC Herman Travers poudly posing on his great adventure.

Despite the unsettled weather, I settled into a daily routine that saw me on the trail at 7 a.m. and in the sleeping bag no later than 9 p.m. As the days gradually grew longer, so did my hours on the trail. With shelters conveniently spaced and a hostel or motel every fourth or fifth night, I was routinely hiking twenty miles a day.

After four nights on the trail, I treated myself to a night at the Relax Inn, a trucker's rest stop with a convenience store and a family-style restaurant. My room, which resembled my college dorm room, was functional cinder block. Like my dorm room, it had a thrift shop TV set on a rickety stand with wheels. Regardless of its appearance, I just hoped the set had a few more hours of life because that night the local PBS affiliate was airing the recently premiered *Alzheimer's Project*, a multimedia production to raise awareness about Alzheimer's disease.

For the next two and a half hours, I was glued to the screen. The first part of the show, "Momentum in Science," dealt with the underlying causes of the disease, current research, and treatment. I quickly learned a lot about neuroanatomy and neuroscience in layman's terms as it pertained to my father's condition.

The second part of the show, "Caregivers," chronicled the lives of five families who faced the daily challenges of the disease. This was not a lesson learned, but a lesson lived. For the next hour, I watched and wept as families like my own struggled to care for their loved ones. Listening to the grieving families, I remembered the day my father stepped into the twilight.

In 2006, two weeks before my parents were to attend my oldest daughter's graduation from the US Coast Guard Academy, my father was hospitalized and evaluated for long-term care at an Alzheimer's facility. That fateful night while watching TV, he turned to my mother with a puzzled look and asked, "Who are you and what are you doing in my house?"

A minute later, he announced that he was "going home" and headed for the front door. My father intended to walk twenty-three miles to his childhood home in the city. Persuading him to stay a little longer, my mother frantically ran to the phone and dialed 911. Minutes later, my father was strapped to a gurney and taken to the hospital. For nearly three years, the family had watched the early symptoms of Alzheimer's advance like gathering storm clouds. Despite the forgetfulness, sporadic confusion, and repetitiveness in his conversation, he remained fairly lucid. To our relief, he did not, nor did he ever, exhibit violent outbursts or threatening behavior. Nevertheless, the day that we had feared had arrived. In layman's terms, the doctor at the hospital said that one of the connectors in his brain had snapped like a rubber band.

The next day when the family visited him, my father repeatedly pleaded with us to take him home in the plaintive voice of a lost child. From the pained expression on my father's face, he obviously knew that something was wrong but was totally clueless. His three-year battle with Alzheimer's had officially begun. He would never come home again nor would he see his granddaughter graduate.

My mother stoically attended graduation because that's what my father would have wanted. Returning home, my mother rallied her flagging spirit and failing health to pursue a new career. Overnight, the nursing home became her personal ministry. She had miraculously transformed a roiling sea of anger into a wellspring of compassion that bubbled pure and sweet from the heart. I marveled at the way she interacted with the staff and residents, comforting, consoling, and befriending every face she met. Like the Energizer Bunny, the "Little Polish Lady" was always on the move, lending a hand in the dining room or talking with the families. With every visit to the nursing home, her prayer list grew longer.

I was not surprised by my mother's response to the disease. Like my father, she was a child of the Depression and tough as nails. When WWII started, she quit her job as a candy maker and became a Rosie the Riveter at the Glenn L. Martin plant where she assembled B-26 bombers. In 1942, while attending a local neighborhood dance, she met a newly minted army lieutenant named Herman Travers. They were married on June 30, 1945. As a new bride, her first challenge was to care for a physically and emotionally wounded veteran who would not be medically discharged from the army until 1947.

Now instead of enjoying the golden years at home with her soul mate, my mother was at my father's side in a life-and-death struggle. The battle would become a soul-searching conflict that shook the foundation of her religious beliefs. "Why does God let these things happen? Your father was a good man," she would often ask me despairingly. I had no answer. Maybe I'd find one on the trail if I kept looking. To do that, I had to keep moving forward one step at a time, and tomorrow promised many more steps.

The next morning as I crossed the Shenandoah Valley, I noticed an unusual chill in the air. That night, temperatures dropped into the mid-30s. The cold was easily manageable in my four-hundred-dollar goose-down sleeping bag, rated at 15 degrees Fahrenheit. The only problem was that I didn't have it. Before leaving

Damascus, I switched my winter bag for a summer bag that was rated at 45 degrees. It didn't seem like a major problem until the "15+" rule was factored. Add 15 degrees to the advertised rating and you'll get the actual rating. I was in bone-chilling and teeth-chattering trouble.

For two nights, I tossed and turned in my sleeping bag while dressed in every piece of clothing that I carried. Sleep came in fitful rounds that lasted an hour or so. No sleep resulted in a tired and grouchy hiker who cursed his stupidity with every step. I had also given my silk sleeping cocoon to Brite. I still had my silk pajama bottoms, but I needed another layer to survive.

In the parking area at US 52, I approached two section hikers who were standing by a red Jeep and explained my situation. "There's a Walmart in the valley. We'll run down there and bring you back. It'll take only a couple of minutes," the driver announced confidently. A minute later, I was firmly wedged in the backseat with a truckload of backpacking gear as Dave sped down the mountain to I-77. Not finding the Walmart or any other store, he headed over another mountain in a different direction.

"Hey, Dave, you'd better slow down, I think your brakes are burning," I shouted over the rush of air. Rounding the next hairpin turn, Dave slowed to a stop and turned on his emergency flashers. All three of us jumped out of the vehicle and ran to the accident scene. A flatbed tractor-trailer with smoke rising from the cab was on its side. About a dozen smashed Harley Davidson motorcycles were scattered on the road. "Jesus, they plowed into a motorcycle gang," I shouted in disbelief. Cautiously approaching the wreckage, we noticed a lot of motorcycle parts on the ground but no bodies or body parts.

"Anybody hurt?" we shouted in unison. There wasn't a moan or groan, only the smell of burning rubber and diesel fuel. Walking behind the trailer, we found two dazed men sitting on the guardrail, nervously smoking cigarettes.

"Brakes gave out coming around the bend. She just flipped and slid along the rail," the one man said.

"We ain't hurt or anything, but it's gonna be a bitch explainin' this to the boss. Guess we were just plain lucky to be alive today," said the other man with a thick southern accent, puffing away furiously. They had been transporting a load of motorcycles to a dealer.

After police and fire personnel arrived, Dave gave a statement to the officer and asked for directions to a clothing store. At a dollar store just off the interstate, I bought the last cotton sweatsuit on the shelf, fire engine red and XXL. Even though the sweats were big and bulky, I couldn't have hiked another day without a good night's sleep. Like the truck drivers, today was my lucky day.

Back in the parking lot, a young couple emerged from the woods as I was stuffing my new pajamas into my backpack. A minute later, William and his wife walked over to me with an insulated cooler bag. "We're done hiking for the day and had some food leftover. You're more than welcome to have what's in the bag," he announced. I repacked to make room for two chicken salad sandwiches, two oranges, and two small bags of potato chips. I emptied my water bottles and refilled them with bottled water.

As we chatted about hiking, I mentioned my rollercoaster ride in search of long underwear. "Don't worry. You only have to suffer for a few more days. The seasonal warm front is arriving to the eastern part of the country later this week. You won't experience any Arctic cold until fall," William assured me with an impish grin.

"Don't tell me you're a weatherman," I joked at the good news.

"No, I'm not a weatherman. I'm a meteorologist with the National Weather Service in Blacksburg," he chuckled.

"That's even better," I replied. "But one nagging question before you leave. If you weather guys can predict the weather, how come you need ten minutes every night on TV and still end up getting it wrong?"

"Sondance, that's not the weather. That's entertainment," he blurted out as the three of us roared with laughter.

That evening at Jenny Knob Shelter, my fellow hikers gawked at my humongous sweats. "It's Clifford," they shouted with laughter, recalling the Big Red Dog from the children's book. But I had the last laugh. The sweats were great for lounging around the shelter and even better for sleeping. Like Floater, I was still a novice hiker who learned another backpacking lesson the hard way. But unlike Floater, I wouldn't have relished Freezer as my new trail name.

I slept soundly for the first time in three nights. Not even the creeping sepulchral layer of cold that drifted along the forest floor at the "Devil's Hour" could disturb my slumber. *All hail King Cotton!* I thought as I wallowed in the warmth. The old backpacking adage that "Cotton Kills" was now "Cotton Thrills."

After two blissful nights of sleep, I walked the streets

of Pearisburg, Virginia, singing "I Love Paris (Pearis)" with Frank Sinatra. After eight days on the trail, I needed a zero day to rest the spirit, heal the body, update the trail journal, and call home. Although Pearisburg had all the hiking conveniences, they were inconveniently stretched out along the main road. The walk from the trail to the Holy Family Hostel, a renovated barn next to the church, was three miles, and no one was willing to give an old altar boy a ride.

The following day, hoping to drum up business for Herm's Hike, I stopped at a nearby nursing home. After speaking with the receptionist, I was directed to an office down the hall. After a few steps, I was blindsided by the smell. Almost daily for the last three years, I had breathed that nauseating aroma of chemical cleaners mixed with traces of urine, feces, and other body odors involved with elder care.

Images of my father's nursing home rushed to my head in a dizzying spiral. My skin turned clammy cold. The walls began to close around me in a blur. Feeling faint, I ran for the front door and didn't stop running until I reached the hostel. Sweating heavily and wheezing, I stumbled to the ground under a shade tree and rested. Except for visiting my father, that was my last visit to a nursing home while on the trail.

That afternoon, I visited the church for some quiet time. I closed my eyes and sat silently in the semidarkness, my mind empty of any thoughts. The intoxicating blend of flowers, burning candles, and a wisp of incense transported me back to my altar boy days at Saint Stanislaus Church. Visions of the Solemn High Mass during Easter and Christmas joyfully danced before me in moments of sheer ecstasy.

Dressed in a red cassock, embroidered white surplice, stiff collar, flourishing silk bowtie, and usually carrying a large candle in a procession, I always felt angelic, waiting for God to personally invite me to his table to break bread with the apostles. With the choir soaring under pulsating rhythm of the heavy-handed pipe organist, I could feel myself rising to the rafters on a mighty cloud of incense.

Later that evening, I walked over to the community room where the pastor, Father John, was holding court for a merry band of parishioners and hikers. A Vietnam veteran with a distinctive New Joisey accent, the jovial priest reminded me of Friar Tuck from the Robin Hood movies in size and demeanor. With an endless supply of snacks and sodas, I spent a delightful evening listening to stories about his former parish in Chincoteague, his uncle the WWII chef, and his ongoing battle over boundary lines with the hospital being built next door. The padre was a skilled raconteur who could rival anyone on the trail. If he ever decided to hike, he could quickly become a trail legend.

On my third day out of Pearisburg, I stopped at the Audie Murphy Monument to pay tribute to America's most-decorated WWII soldier. On May 28, 1971, Murphy's plane crashed nearby into the side of Brush Mountain. The poster boy for America's fighting men was dead at the age of forty-five.

After placing a small rock on the large cairn next to the monument, an angled chunk of engraved granite, I sat on the bench to reminisce about my father.

If there was ever a poster boy for the Greatest

Generation, it was my dad. Dropping out of high school in the ninth grade during the Great Depression, he found a job to support the family at one of the "packing houses" that lined Baltimore's waterfront. Hours were long, wages were short, and working conditions deplorable as seasonal fruit and vegetables were cleaned, steamed, canned, and shipped.

A few years later when the next eldest sibling found work, my father was free to follow his dream. His journey began with a long walk to the recruiter's office in downtown Baltimore. Rejected by the navy for bad teeth and the marines for bad feet, he ironically joined the army as an infantryman. Racing home, he packed a small duffel bag and headed out the door for an adventure of a lifetime in the tropical paradise of Hawaii.

Promoted to private first class as the outstanding recruit in basic training, my father was assigned to the 27th Infantry Regiment at Schofield Barracks. He had found a calling in the army and a home with the Wolfhounds, whose regimental life was the background for the novel and movie *From Here to Eternity*. At breakfast on the morning of December 7, 1941, he witnessed Japanese dive-bombers roaring overhead on their way to Pearl Harbor and fired some of the first shots of the war. Following the attack, he was assigned to patrol duty along Waikiki Beach. His calling was now a call to arms that grew louder with each day.

Commissioned in late 1942 as a second lieutenant, he returned to the Pacific Campaign with the 323rd Regimental Combat Team and fought alongside the marines at the Battle of Peleliu. On that remote coral island, known as the Antietam of the Pacific for its bloody and brutal skirmishes, his courage was put to the ultimate test. On the evening of October 17, 1944, he successfully led a team of volunteers to rescue wounded men who were stranded on the battlefield. Deadly enemy mortar killed one of his men and wounded another, but four soldiers were dragged from the kill zone to safety. Two weeks later on October 30, while on patrol near Bloody Nose Ridge, he was seriously wounded while directing a counterattack after being ambushed by withering enemy machine-gun fire. The bullet had nearly severed his foot below the ankle. Walking, especially long distances, would never be his stock-in-trade.

Sent back to the States, my father spent the next two years in and out of military hospitals before being discharged in 1947. A lover of the outdoors, his dream of a career as a state trooper, a park policeman, or even a mailman was scuttled by his war injury. Seeking job security for his family, he worked for thirty-two years as a window clerk for the US Post Office.

Like Murphy, my father received a number of medals for heroism in combat and a Purple Heart. Unlike Murphy, who became a Hollywood star, my father remained an unsung hero, a distinction of honor that would be passed down to his children and grandchildren. Before leaving, I placed another stone on the cairn in honor of my father. I wondered if my father's life would have turned out differently if he had had a chance to walk off the war like Earl Shaffer, the first man to thru-hike the AT in 1948. Instead of walking off the war, my father returned home to work off the war.

Rummaging through my backpack, I found my father's dog tag that I had been carrying as a good-luck charm and tied it around my neck with a piece of string. I was now walking off the war for my father. If not for my father's love, I could have easily been walking off the war for both of us. Having seen the horrors of war up close, my father made me promise in 1969 that I would graduate from college before entertaining any ideas about joining the military. He didn't want to see an academic scholarship wasted or see his oldest son slaughtered on the battlefield. I saw his troubled heart with compassion and kept my promise, becoming the first college graduate on either side of the family.

After a leisurely afternoon, I picked up the pace, stopping briefly for photos at a rock formation known as the Dragon's Tooth. My goal was dinner at the Homeplace in Catawba. Since Pearisburg, hikers had been raving about the converted old farmhouse that served the best fried chicken in the South with an AYCE buffet. My mouth watered at the thought.

Minutes later, any ideas about a speed hike were literally dashed against rocks. The climb down the mountain included a rock wall with rebar handrails. After mulling over my options, which included simply throwing myself off the cliff, I pulled out the cord for my food bag and gently lowered my backpack to the ground before descending inch by inch.

By the time I arrived at the front door of the restaurant, it was closed. While standing in the parking lot, looking forlorn at the prospect of a freeze-dried dinner, a pickup truck with Marine Corps stickers across the rear bumper pulled up next to me. Jesse, the bearded and ponytailed driver, offered a place to camp and a dinner. Earlier he had corralled the Stooges, three young men from Holland who had the honor of leading the parade at the Trail Days.

That evening while dining on beer, pizza, and apple pie, Jesse regaled us with stories about his childhood and his tour of duty in Vietnam with a covert recon unit, elaborating on his famous "death punch" that could stop a beating heart. Thankfully, he didn't ask for any volunteers. After breakfast the next morning, Jesse drove me back to the trail to slackpack for the day.

I was reluctant to leave my backpack with a stranger, but if I couldn't trust a fellow marine then whom could I trust? Four miles up the trail, I stopped at the iconic McAfee Knob, a rock ledge jutting from the top of a cliff like a diving board. On this Saturday afternoon before Memorial Day, the knob was crawling with day hikers and young children. To get my quintessential Kodak moment on the ledge, I had to wait in line.

Miles later, I traversed Tinker Cliffs. The sandstone outcropping that extended for nearly half a mile was reportedly named for the large number of Revolutionary War deserters, tinkers by trade, who hid in the area. With its maze of crevices and caves, the cliffs would have made an excellent hiding place. Farther along, I saw my first sign of impending civilization. Hay Rock was covered in spray-painted graffiti.

As I headed down the last mountain of the day, I crossed Tinker Creek on a one-lane, abandoned, concrete bridge. The creek was made famous by American author Annie Dillard in her 1974 book *Pilgrim at Tinker Creek*. A contemporary heir to Henry David Thoreau and the Transcendentalist movement, Dillard chronicled a year of exploration, contemplation, and inspiration in the natural world at the creek.

Being an ardent disciple of "Uncle Hank," as I affectionately called Mr. Thoreau, I stopped for a meditative moment. Gazing downstream, I wondered how many of my fellow hikers realized the significance of this narrow ribbon of shallow water that lazily flowed toward the Dillard homestead. At the creek's edge, I stepped into the holy water and let it flow around the soles of my boots. I knew that Annie would understand the meaning of this symbolic gesture.

A half-mile up the trail, I stopped at US 220 to end the day's journey. About fifty yards to my right was the Howard Johnson hotel that Jesse promised. I entered the small lobby and stood behind a man who was engaged in an escalating argument with the Pakistani desk clerk about money and cigarettes that were missing from his room. The man, whom I had seen earlier on the trail, had the creepy and cunning appearance of Charles Manson. He was a red flag hiker to be avoided at all costs. I stepped to the side and waited for him to leave.

After securing one of the last rooms, I presented my credit card and driver's license. "Are you *the* Paul Travers?" the woman asked expectantly.

"I believe I am," I replied somewhat confused, wondering how many of me were staying at the hotel.

"Then I believe these belong to you," she said pointing to my backpack and a brown paper bag on the floor behind the counter. I retrieved my pack and peeked inside the bag. The six-pack of beer was still cold.

After a quick shower, I grabbed the bag and strolled over to the pool to soak my feet. To my utter delight, the pool was overrun with beer and bikinis. The hotel was headquarters for a holiday weekend softball tournament.

"Jesse, this Bud's for you," I declared joyfully, popping one of the cans and lifting it to the sky. True to the creed, marines took care of their own in beer and battle.

Except for witnessing the abhorrent argument at the front desk that evolved into racial and ethnic slurs from the allegedly aggrieved hiker, it had been a day filled with sunshine and spectacular overlooks. The vigil at Tinker Creek had been icing on the cake.

Even though it had been over thirty years since I read Dillard's book, her thought-provoking narrative embodied many of my personal beliefs. Like Dillard, I first encountered Thoreau and his literary companions Walt Whitman and Ralph Waldo Emerson in a high school English class. Although I wasn't able to fully grasp all of their philosophical treatises at the time, their writings had me thinking about my own life.

I had grown in the era of peace and love that was exemplified by hippies, yippies, peaceniks, beatniks, the Vietnam War, and Woodstock. Introducing the Transcendentalists, who questioned the rigid values of the status quo in politics and religion, to a boys' Catholic high school was risky. I don't think teachers realized they were playing with fire, and some of the students were walking the hallways with sticks of dynamite in their heads. The counterculture was talking about my generation, and I was listening. I hoped that one of the poolside boom boxes would crank out our cultural anthem, The Who's "My Generation."

Chapter 13
Death of a Hollywood Starlet
(Daleville to Waynesboro, VA)

Before leaving the motel, I declined an invite from one of the teams to watch the tournament with a promise of more beer and bikinis. There might even be a chance to play if I wanted. For an old player that was a tempting offer, but I held firm. The crowd at the motel was simply driving me crazy. I craved the peace and quiet of the woods. In another three days, a motel was waiting in the town of Glasgow. With a forecast of sunny skies with intermittent showers, I couldn't afford to stay away from nature's playground, my current place of employment.

A few miles from the motel, I walked under I-81 and crossed the Shenandoah Valley. For the next ten miles, I slowly ascended the spine of the Blue Ridge Mountains. For the next one hundred fifty miles, the trail intertwined with the Blue Ridge Parkway until it reached the town of Waynesboro, Virginia, where it became the famous Skyline Drive.

Due to my late start from the Sunday breakfast buffet, I arrived at the Montvale Overlook before dusk. In the fading light, distant mountains were flaunting their characteristic blue haze. While enjoying the view of

Goose Creek Valley, a car pulled into the parking lot. Out stepped an older couple, somewhere in their seventies, who took a few pictures. Seeing my backpack, they walked over to talk.

"How so?" the man inquired intently when I referred to the hike as my spiritual journey.

"I think God is following me on the trail," I chuckled after telling my story about the angel at Clingmans Dome and the prayer session at Damascus.

"Did you ever think that God is leading?" the man responded, reaching for his wallet. With a mischievous grin, he handed me his business card: Reverend Wayne L. Reed, Pastor - Snellville Congregational Methodist Church.

"Well, it looks like this proves my theory about God following. Maybe he should be walking alongside me," I kidded.

"I think he already is," Reverend Reed chuckled. After delivering a brief history of Herm's Hike, the couple, who were visiting a church in the area, offered me a few candy bars and a bottle of fruit juice. We then joined hands and prayed for my hike, my parents, and the rest of the hikers on the trail. "If you ever get down to Georgia again, look us up. We'd love to have you at our service," the reverend announced before getting into his car.

I arrived at the nondescript Bobblets Gap Shelter hoping the shelter sign would read Heaven's Gate, Angel's Loft, or something spiritual. But instead of working on signs, God had taken the day off and was busy walking with me. The next morning at breakfast, a southbound section hiker (SOBO) was raving about the best hamburger on the trail. "Fresh ground beef made to order," he boasted.

"Lead me into temptation," I cackled as I jotted down the directions.

Late that morning as instructed, I walked down a gravel road that supposedly led to the Middle Creek Campground. After about a mile, I stopped and reassessed my appetite. I hadn't seen a road sign or marker since I left the trail. Not wanting to waste any more energy in the heat of the day, I headed back to the trail. Halfway up the hill, a decrepit vehicle pulled alongside me. The driver, who appeared to be in his late seventies or early eighties, was behind the wheel of a Ford sedan from the late '70s or early '80s. After mentioning my search for the elusive campground, the driver motioned for me to get in.

"Name's Roy," the driver said, extending a thick, meaty hand. "I'm out for my weekly drive and wouldn't mind some company if you got the time."

"As long as we get to the campground for lunch, I'm game," I replied, not wanting to disappoint my trail angel. For the next hour, Roy drove the country roads with a steady monologue about his life. Along the way, he pointed out personal landmarks, such as the house where he lived, the schoolhouse where he studied, and the farm where he worked. It was a fascinating history lesson about a man and his times in bygone Appalachia.

"Ran away from home to join the circus and ended up joining the army. Came back home, did some logging before buying a farm. Hard work with little pay, but it beat the hell of going down a coal mine. Always liked being outdoors. Right now, I'm living with my daughter, but she wants me to start thinking about a retirement home. I'm thinking about running away again. Guess I'll have to wait until the circus comes to town," he laughed at the irony of his joke.

"Roy, I know how you feel. A retirement home is not necessarily a home away from home," I said sympathetically before telling him the story about my father.

"Well, Paul, then you do know how I feel." Roy frowned.

Pulling up to the campground office, Roy reached for his wallet and handed me a ten-dollar bill for Herm's Hike. I thanked Roy for his donation and wondered who would be his next history student. All it took was a little wandering.

Inside the small luncheonette, Susan, the owner, was busy thawing out a mound of ground beef. After feasting on two of the freshest hamburgers on the trail, she drove me back to the trailhead. "Be careful out there. Heavy thunderstorms due this afternoon," she warned.

Susan's forecast was accurate. Two miles down the trail, the skies opened with a torrential downpour. I frantically pulled out the rain cover for my pack and donned my rain jacket. In the steep climb up Fork Mountain, I was sweating heavily and getting soaked inside and out. Finding a clump of trees, I waited out the storm under an umbrella of dripping leaves.

Two miles later, under a burning sun, I arrived at Bryant Ridge Shelter. The new, tri-level, timber-framed structure with Plexiglas windows that slept twenty was an architectural wonder and one of the finest shelters on the trail. With more dark clouds on the horizon, it seemed like the perfect place to take a nap in the midday heat. Stepping inside to inspect the premises, I quickly changed my mind.

On the first floor, a sick hiker was curled up in a sleeping bag, moaning and squirming in pain. Now I knew why his friends were milling around outside and talking in hushed tones. When I told them about the nearby campground, they said their friend was going to wait a day or two to see if the malady passed. Thinking Hantavirus, hepatitis, or the bubonic plague, I decided not to wait. The next shelter was only four miles away.

As I was leaving, two more hikers arrived on the scene. One was a tall, ruggedly built middle-aged man with white hair while the other was a much shorter and younger man with dark hair. They went inside and returned a few minutes later. I overheard them telling the hiker's friends that they were willing to carry their friend back to the main road. When the offer was declined, the Good Samaritans walked over to me and introduced themselves. "I'm Circuit Rider and this is my partner Sherlock," the older man said, extending his hand.

"Don't tell me, you're a man of the cloth," I chuckled.

"How did you guess?" he asked with surprise. "Not too many people pick up on the history of the name."

"Reverend, I've seen all the Clint Eastwood westerns, *Lonesome Dove*, and *Deadwood*," I boasted. I was more than familiar with the riding clergymen, mostly Baptist and Methodist, who brought religion to the isolated settlements in Appalachia and later the Wild West.

Since 1991, Bill Newman (Circuit Rider) and Henri Aldunate (Sherlock) had been hiking the AT to provide emotional, physical, and spiritual aid to hikers. Originally associated with a Baptist church in Michigan, the pastor and his youth leader had developed a trail ministry named Heartbeat Appalachian Trail.

When the conversation shifted to my father's battle with Alzheimer's, I told them the ordeal had been extremely hard on my mother's faith in God. They quickly decided to remedy the situation. As the sun disappeared behind a bank of menacing clouds, the three of us held hands and prayed.

"Heavenly Father, we call on you today as God the Great Physician to heal the heart of Paul's mother," Circuit Rider implored tenderly. "Bind up her spiritual wounds and give her spirit the strength to care for her loving husband. We also ask that you shine your healing grace on Paul and his family. This we ask from your humble servants. Amen."

Tears flowed down my cheeks in response to those impassioned words as I thought about my mother. She had always prayed for others. Now it was time to pray for her. I hoped that hundreds of miles away she felt her soul instilled with an inner peace. It certainly uplifted my spirit. Without a doubt, Baptists and Methodists were the masters of the impromptu prayer. It was nothing like the scripted Hail Mary and Our Father bromides from my Catholic upbringing when priests made prayer a penance. After complimenting my prayer group, they laughed in agreement. "There's plenty of prayers waiting for you, Sondance," Circuit Rider added. "The mountain spring that gushes from the heart never runs dry."

Circuit Rider and Sherlock quickly took their leave and headed up the trail as thunder boomed overhead. Seconds later, I heard the rain blowing through the trees with a frightening sizzle. When a blinding flash of light exploded on the ridge behind me like a white phosphorous shell, I took evasive action. I immediately sprinted after the pair, thinking it would be better to be struck down by lightning with two men of the cloth than by myself. If anyone could pray his way into heaven, it was Circuit Rider. I would be listening intently as he stated his case, making sure he mentioned my name.

The next morning, I crossed Apple Orchard Mountain. From 1955 to 1974, the US Air Force operated a radar station on the summit that included barracks for 120 men, several Quonset huts for radar equipment, and a concrete bomb shelter. Today all that stood was a radar dome operated by the Federal Aviation Administration and a couple of service buildings surrounded by barbed-wire fence. At 4,225 feet, the mountain was the highest point on the trail until I reached Mount Moosilauke in New Hampshire more than a thousand miles away. However, that didn't mean there weren't any hard climbs between the two points. Hiking up a thousand feet in a mile was the same, regardless if you started at sea level or Everest base camp.

The next day after a fast and furious nine-mile hike from High Knob, I crossed the James River on the James River Foot Bridge, the longest pedestrian bridge on the trail at 623 feet. Dedicated to the memory of Bill Foot, a 1987 thru-hiker who spearheaded the effort to build the walkway on old railroad piers, it spawned a dangerous tradition. But today with the murky river running high and fast and tree limbs spinning madly in the current, there would be no daredevil hikers making the jump.

Ready for my "nero" day, I hitched a ride into Glasgow. Unfortunately, the town wasn't ready for me.

The motel had closed three months earlier, too late to be updated in my trail companion. The good news was that town officials were providing camping space behind the firehouse. With a supermarket and dollar store nearby, I decided to spend the night.

That afternoon in the town park, I emptied my backpack and dried out everything on the aluminum bleachers at the softball field. A flyer on a bulletin board announced tonight's game between the town of Glasgow and the Glasgow VFD. If it didn't rain, I had a free ball game and the best seat in the ballpark.

At around 4 o'clock, two of the players, a town employee nicknamed Hammer and a young gentleman with special needs named Dustin, began sprucing up the field for the game. They meticulously mowed the grass, raked the infield, painted foul lines, and cleaned the bases.

Being the only spectator, I struck up a conversation with the men. "I can't make it tonight. If you want to play, be here at around 5 o'clock. Dustin will take care of everything for you," Hammer announced.

"I'll be right here until tomorrow morning," I replied enthusiastically. I jumped at the chance even though it had been thirty years since I played in a league softball game.

The game started at 6 o'clock right after the playing of the national anthem. The stands were packed with friends and family members. I was in the starting line-up for the fire department, batting tenth and playing right center field. Under the discerning eyes of my teammates, I warmed up stiffly. From their looks, they were wondering if this senior thru-hiker could still play ball, and so was I.

To secure a spot in the starting line-up, I bragged

that I could roll out of my sleeping bag and line a single to center. And that's exactly what I did, not once but twice. I went 2 for 3 (two line-drive singles) with a walk and a sacrifice fly. While my swing was sweet, my feet were rusty. Running around the bases after 775 miles on the trail was not easy or pretty. My boots felt like they had lead soles.

Late in the game when I was at the plate with runners on base, the crowd started chanting. "Sondance! Sondance," they yelled as they stomped the bleachers with a metallic rumble. I stepped out of the batter's box and tipped my visor cap to my fans. How I loved Glasgow! We won 13 to 11 after being down by 6 runs in the third inning. Dustin played the last three innings and slapped an RBI single through the infield. It was a great night for baseball! It was a great night for an old catcher!

Following the game, everyone shared a few beers. I thanked both teams for allowing me the chance to recapture my youth if only for a couple of hours. As the crowd headed for their cars, someone flipped the light switch. The ballpark fell dark and quiet. I sat alone in the bleachers, stared at the empty field, and smiled. I had to be the only hiker in AT history looking for trail magic on a field of dreams that vanished over forty years ago. The crazy thing was that I found it.

That evening, I walked to centerfield and disappeared in the darkness as if I were walking into the fictional cornfield from the movie *Field of Dreams*. My home was the gazebo and my bed was the picnic table with a mattress of cardboard boxes that I fished out of a dumpster. As thunderstorms raced across the valley, I slept comfortably dry, protected by a wall of overturned picnic tables. The only casualty was my sweatsuit that I absentmindedly left on one of the benches. Saturated with water, it weighed around five pounds. I wrung it out, folded it neatly, and left it on the bench. I didn't need it any longer. The weather had broken as predicted.

After Glasgow, it was three good hiking days to the next hostel. For the last day's seventeen-mile hike from Buena Vista to Montebello, I had good weather, a good path, great scenery, and a great hiking companion. Snowhead, one of the trail's greyhounds, was finishing a section hike. We ended the day at the trailhead where he had a cooler of cold beer in the trunk of his car.

I spent the night at the Dutch Haus in the town of Montebello. The log cabin home and adjoining log cabin bunkhouse were the epitome of trail luxury that featured the luxurious Dutch Haus bathrobe. For a ridiculously low rate, I had a private room, a home-cooked dinner of stuffed peppers, a gourmet breakfast, and the gracious company of the owners Earl and Lois.

During dessert that evening, we introduced ourselves around the table and talked about our hikes. We were all over forty, an oddity on the trail, with a wealth of life experiences. After everyone had finished their monologue, one of the hikers, whom I did not recognize, started the interrogation.

"Are you the guy that claims he was wanted by the FBI?" the man chided. When I told that I was, he badgered me with questions about the incident. When I told him about the cover-up at my former place of employment, he grew agitated. "I worked for the FBI for over twenty-five years and never heard of such nonsense."

"Obviously, you didn't get out of the office too

much during your career," I scoffed. "Just take a look at whistleblowers from the Vietnam War to the present. And I know because I witnessed one of those cover-ups." All heads now looked at me with quizzical, furrowed brows. It was time to put up or shut up.

"Does anyone remember Buffy, the child actress, from the TV show *Family Affair* in the late '60s and early '70s?" I asked my audience.

"Yeah, she died from a drug overdose," someone replied.

"Exactly, but she didn't die where the authorities said she died," I surmised coyly. "The tabloids and the coroner's office reported that she died at a crash pad in Oceanside, California, but she actually died at the bachelor officer quarters (BOQ) on the Marine Corps base at Camp Pendleton." I lowered my voice for dramatic effect and solved one of Hollywood's great mysteries.

The following statement is what I witnessed and what I believe happened

On August 28, 1976, I was officer of the day (OD) at the Delmar Area, part of the base located along the Pacific Ocean and adjacent to the town of Oceanside. After making my rounds at 3 o'clock on that Saturday morning, I instructed my jeep driver to take me to the nearby BOQ so I could pick up a change of clothes.

Nothing was unusual at the complex except for the ambulance parked in front of the building. As I walked over to the vehicle, a clanging sound pierced the stillness. Two ambulance attendants were coming down the outside stairwell of the building with a gurney. When they stopped to open the back doors to the ambulance, I couldn't help but notice a white sheet covering a petite body.

"Do you mind telling me what's going on here?" I demanded, introducing myself as the OD and stepping next to the gurney. The attendants looked nervously at each other.

"Sorry, Lieutenant, but we can't help you. We're under strict orders not to talk or stop for anyone," one of the attendants stated. I slowly lifted the top sheet on the gurney and saw strands of blonde hair. "Lieutenant, I wouldn't do that if I were you," the attendant admonished, yanking my hand away from the sheet.

Without another word, the attendants quickly loaded the gurney and disappeared silently into the night like grave robbers. The attendants had refused to give me their names, but I took down the license plate number on the ambulance.

Hurrying inside to the registration desk, I asked the duty NCO (noncommissioned officer) if she knew what had happened. Sarge, whom I had known since my first day on the base, directed me to her office and closed the door. "Lieutenant, take my advice. You didn't see anything here tonight. Just forget about it and don't go around asking any questions because nobody is going to answer them, including me."

I returned to battalion headquarters and filled out the daily log, noting the time and place of the incident with a brief description. The following Monday morning I was ordered to report to the commander's office. Behind closed doors, the colonel questioned me about the event and handed me the OD logbook. My entry had been removed, and a new sheet had been inserted that made no mention of the incident. I was instructed to sign the logbook, which I did without question or comment, and ordered not to discuss this alleged incident with anyone unless directed by higher command.

Once outside I ran over to the PX to get a newspaper. The front page reported that TV actress Anissa Jones, age eighteen, had been found dead in an Oceanside bungalow from an apparent drug overdose. Back at the BOQ, I checked with friends who lived near the stairwell. No one heard or saw a thing. However, the two junior officers with a suite on that floor had vanished. Their room was empty. Scuttlebutt reported that Jones had been doing drugs earlier that day with a group of marines and the party eventually moved to the BOQ. I didn't know where the party started, but I definitely knew where it ended.

Later that evening, a fellow hiker cornered me about my inquisitor. "His trail name is Hoover, and he's the biggest ass you'd ever want to meet. And, by the way, that's one of the best stories I heard on the trail." I was slowly developing a cult following.

Before I could think about Waynesboro and a long-awaited break, I had some difficult hiking ahead of me for the next two and a half days. At Priest Shelter, hikers confess their real or imaginary sins in the logbook with comic flair much to the delight of readers. Eschewing the traditional confession, I assumed my earlier persona of "Paul on the Road to Damascus" and wrote the following: "A reading from a letter of Paul to the Appalachians. Brothers and sisters, let us go forth to the mountains and seek spiritual refuge in its peaks. Let these holy places nourish the soul and reflect the goodness and greatness of God." I had heard the call of the sacred mountains and was ready to preach the word of Appalachian salvation.

Just beyond the shelter, I caught up with Mother Nature, one of the dinner guests at Dutch Haus, who was section hiking. The petite former physical education teacher in her mid-sixties was a fellow graduate from the University of Maryland. We had a common bond that we were eagerly willing to share. The tough miles passed unnoticed in hilarious revelry as we swapped college stories. Both of us had attended college against the backdrop of the movie *Animal House* as spectators and participants. Although she graduated in 1967, six years ahead of me, the debauchery and depravity remained the same. About the only things that changed were the hairstyles and wardrobes.

A few years ago, she had remarried her first husband, whom she had met in college, after her second husband passed away. Despite the romantic notion of your first true love, she wasn't quite sure if that was true the second time around. And that's the reason why she was on the trail. She hoped her wilderness sojourn would mediate her amorous dilemma. It was another love story with a different twist to add to my collection.

Mother Nature, true to her name, was a free spirit. Taking breaks at scenic overlooks, we always broke out in song before returning to the trail. Unabashedly, we sang to the glory of the mountains that stretched before us. Our song list was short but sweet. It included "America the Beautiful" and "God Bless America" along with a few tunes from the Beatles and Bob Dylan. We ended each performance with a rendition of "Wild Thing."

On the last day into Waynesboro, we hiked over twenty miles with a young female hiker named Creek

Dancer. By the end of the day, I was gassed. It wasn't the distance; it was the speed that was killing me. Struggling to maintain the pace and my pride, it was painfully obvious that old age had caught up with me. My days of chasing fast women, any women for that matter, were ancient history.

That evening, the three of us dined at an AYCE Chinese buffet. Before leaving, I picked up a handful of fortune cookies, ever so curious to see what they would say about the coming week, a week that I had been awaiting anxiously since Springer Mountain.

After a restful night at the Grace Evangelical Lutheran Church, I took my long-awaited zero day. With showers, snacks, and movies, the hostel was a great place for R&R. When my brother Mark arrived the following morning to hike, I was ready for another curious adventure. My spiritual journey had become a magical mystery tour that was patiently waiting to take me away once again. My collection of fortune cookies, an edible AT crystal ball, could attest to that belief. One of them from the previous night read, "You are in for an enlightening experience." I couldn't wait to hike or open the next cookie. The healing power of the mountains was waiting to be tested.

Chapter 14
Ode to a Mountain Poet
(Waynesboro to Pen Mar Park, MD)

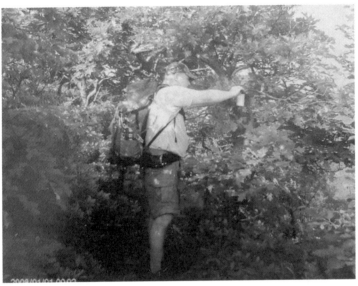

My brother Mark, The Postmaster, honors his son, a mountain poet.

Our first order of business in Shenandoah National Park was to self-register at the park's kiosk, a subtle reminder that Big Brother was watching our every move. Back home, I was certain my phone was being tapped by the feds. With Mark being a novice hiker, we decided that our daily mileage would be twelve to fourteen miles. That plan was immediately scuttled. The first shelter was twenty miles up the trail. After a thirteen-mile day, we stealth camped at a scenic overlook off the highway. One day on the trail, and we were already outlaws. I wondered if the feds were watching us from a spy satellite.

The second night we found the law and the Lord at the Loft Mountain Campground. While deer browsed our campsite, Mark and I crawled on our hands and knees frantically searching for my green coin purse that contained money, credit card, health card, and driver's license.

"Don't worry. You'll find it in the morning," Mark reassured me as we crawled into our tents. "I'll say a prayer to Saint Anthony," he chuckled.

"What's he going to do? Show up here tomorrow morning and help us look?" I replied sarcastically.

I fumed at my stupidity. The money could easily be replaced, but the cards could not. If I didn't find the purse, I'd have to get off the trail and get new ones. The bureaucratic hassle could take time that we didn't have. My brother and I had just spent two enjoyable days swapping stories and sharing memories from our childhood days. If I had to get off the trail, the hike for my brother was over. He only had a week off from work. In one last futile attempt, I backtracked along the asphalt road to the campground office with my headlamp. All I found in the night was thirty-five cents in change, a dime and a quarter.

Early the following morning, I slowly crawled out of my tent in the semidarkness to heed the call of nature. Beyond the tent canopy, my hand landed on something soft and lumpy. I had found my purse. I shook my head with a tight grin. Mark and I had searched every inch of ground around my tent a couple of times. I could only conclude that Saint Anthony had good night vision.

The next day we stopped at Hightop Hut so Mark could experience shelter life. It was an experience he'd never forget. After securing space in the shelter, we stood under the canopy and watched the parade of hikers come in from the rain. Dripping wet, one hiker dropped his backpack in front of the shelter and pulled out a rain jacket. "I didn't think the rain would be this wet," he declared, zipping up the jacket. Mark looked at me, tilted his head toward the hiker, and grinned. He had heard the story. I smiled and nodded, stifling a laugh. Mojo had arrived.

I first met Mojo while hiking from Daleville. He was sitting on a rock beside the trail carefully rolling a joint, which he politely offered to share. I politely declined. That evening at the shelter, he decided to relax with a toke, but first he needed a light and nobody had a lighter. After fumbling with a couple of damp matches, the matchbook suddenly erupted into flames. With a flick of a wrist, he tossed the flaming chunk of cardboard into the shelter where it landed on top of a sleeping bag.

Fearing the shelter would erupt in a fireball, hikers pounced on the smoldering bag. In a flash of rage, the bag's owner, a rather large, bearded hiker who looked more like a large, bearded biker, dashed across the floor. With one hand, he pinned Mojo against the wall and raised a fist. Before any blows could be struck, he was bear hugged by one of his friends.

"You stupid shit. You owe me a new sleeping bag," the hiker screamed angrily as spittle flew from his mouth. "Get the fuck out here before I smash your face."

"Hey, man, I'm good for it," Mojo replied, his hands trembling. Without another word, he picked up his joint, grabbed his backpack, and disappeared into the woods. I had hoped that I had seen the last of another red flag hiker, but a week later he was back.

At dinner that evening, Mojo grumbled that no one in Waynesboro would sell him marijuana because they thought he was an undercover narcotics officer with his short hair. That comment got the ball rolling. Throughout the evening, he regaled us with his comic adventures in pursuit of white blazes and nickel bags. My brother and I laughed until we cried. Mojo should have been hiking with Cheech and Chong.

At breakfast the next day, a hiker asked Mark his trail name. When he said that he didn't have one, the hiker asked him what he did for a living. "I work for the Postal Service," my brother replied.

"Oh, so you're a postmaster?"

"No, I buy equipment," Mark responded.

"Well, you look like a postmaster to me," the hiker quipped. A backhanded comment or not, a great trail name had been born. Unlike me, it only took him three days to find it.

We hiked a short distance to the rocky outcropping at Hightop Mountain. With its stunning views in the early morning light, it was the perfect spot to begin our memorial tribute to Justin. Mark's youngest son had been tragically killed in a handgun accident at the age of twelve.

For seven years, my brother and his wife had been living every parent's worst nightmare. There was some consolation with the harvesting of organs for needy recipients, but the sorrow was overwhelming. Following the funeral, my brother's personality changed in subtle ways. Not surprisingly the twinkle in his eyes had dimmed; the smile had slightly soured. Years later, my mother confided that it was the same changes that she had witnessed with my father when he returned from the war. Like my father, my brother weaved the pain into the fabric of his life and moved forward. Today moving forward meant scaling a mountain to honor his son. The hike was now dedicated to a higher calling, Herman and Justin.

Reaching into his backpack, the Postmaster retrieved a bag of poems. Written by Justin, they were printed on rectangular slips of green paper with paper ties. From the age of ten until his death, the precocious poet had written a volume of poetry that expounded on life and love against a background of clouds, mountains, oceans, trees, and anything that nature had to offer. Each of us grabbed a handful of poems and hung them on the adjacent trees like Christmas ornaments. When we finished, poems twisted and turned in the breeze like Tibetan prayer flags. I had no doubt the trees were honored to sing the praises of this unsung poet. We continued the tribute at every suitable mountaintop along Skyline Drive.

After four days on the trail, I was confident that Postmaster was ready to face the ultimate trail challenge, two nights of comfort and cooked meals. To celebrate our success on the trail, we spent the night at Big Meadows Lodge where we shared a room, something we hadn't done since we were kids. The following night we stayed at Skyland and shared a cabin. Our timing was impeccable.

Both nights, severe thunderstorms rolled over the mountains with heavy rain and lightning.

At Skyland's dining room, we struck up a conversation with a retired couple who had been day hiking. "Just the other day we discovered a body next to the trail. The young man said he was taking a nap, but he was passed out cold next to a pile of beer cans," the woman groused. "I believe his name was Ho-Ho or something like that."

"Mojo," Mark and I shouted in laughter.

"Yes, I believe that was it," the lady replied curtly. The couple was not amused with our story of the wayward hiker. They couldn't understand how a young man could hike his way to Maine under the influence of alcohol and drugs, and neither could we.

For the next three days, we continued to covertly post Justin's poems. Our efforts did not go unnoticed. At the shelters, we often heard hikers talking about the green tags hanging from the trees. Upon first sight, many hikers thought the poems were dollar bills placed by a trail angel. "Who was this mystery poet?" they wondered aloud. My brother and I just nodded our heads in agreement and smiled, content to keep the mystery a secret.

While having lunch at the Elkwallow Wayside on our penultimate day, we spotted Mojo on the patio. His shirt was covered oddly in black dots. After eating, we ambled over to his table for a hiking update. We couldn't resist the temptation.

"I'm up to thirty-four," he proudly boasted as he swatted another fly. When I told him about the couple at Skyland, he confirmed their story. "Bought a six-pack for later that night, but it was too heavy to carry so I decided to drink it on the trail. With the heat and the other stuff, I passed out."

Postmaster and I wished him well and hightailed it up the trail. "At least, we solved the mystery of the black spots," I chuckled.

"He smelled like road kill," Postmaster bellowed. "Instead of flies, there should have been maggots." To our relief, Mojo didn't stay at the shelter that evening. To my relief, I never saw him again.

The next day Mark's son picked us up at Front Royal and drove us to my brother's home in nearby Manassas. That evening at a cookout, some of Mark's friends commented to me that they hadn't seen him this relaxed since Justin's death. While taking breaks from the onslaught of beef and beer, I frequently gazed over where Postmaster was holding court with his guests. I couldn't help but notice the broad smile and the twinkle in his eye as he relived his trail adventures.

My brother had far exceeded my expectations as a hiker. It's not easy to step away from a desk, shoulder your backpack, and hike a hundred mountain miles on the AT. Despite the PUDS and sore knees, the former army officer, who played college football as a defensive lineman, soldiered on without complaint. I told him that he should be proud of his accomplishment. Anytime he wanted to hike, just call. The Postmaster didn't have to ring twice.

At the trailhead the following morning, Postmaster handed me a bag of food and a bag of poems, a gentle reminder there were many more mountains to decorate. I meandered along the trail thinking about my nephew. His poems now lived in the Blue Ridge Mountains like stained-glass windows in a gothic cathedral. As I walked in silence, I experienced another religious epiphany. The great stone cathedrals of the world were man's attempt to recreate mountaintops. There was no finer tribute to God or Justin.

I then remembered my own personal tribute to my nephew. When my brother and his wife were deciding on a gravestone, they had mentioned the possibility of an inscription. After searching futilely for a befitting poem, I tried my own hand. Everyone loved it, including the stonemason who was so moved that he inscribed the following words for free: "Goodbye, sweet poet. Go gently in the night. For on the distant horizon, there is the dawn of a new tomorrow where we will meet again." I took some literary satisfaction in knowing that my words had been immortalized in granite. They had become part of a mountain.

For the next three days, I hiked with a heightened sense of anticipation. Harper's Ferry, the psychological halfway point, was only fifty miles away. I was getting closer to home with each step. After a night at the dilapidated plywood configuration named Dick's Dome Shelter, I endured a strenuous eighteen-mile day.

After a delightful sunny stroll through the wildflowers at Sky Meadows State Park, the day ended with a punishing climb to the backdoor of the Bear's Den hostel. My nemesis at midpoint was the Rollercoaster, a thirteen-and-a-half-mile section of steep, rocky terrain with loose rocks.

The trail "ride" was a stroke of marketing genius by the local trail club. When you don't have a trail, simply put up a sign with a catchy name and challenge hikers.

At the start, there was a warning sign in bold, capital letters that read "Hiker Notice – Warning!! You are about to enter The Rollercoaster. Built and maintained by the 'Trailboss' and his merry crew of volunteers. Have a great ride and we will see you at the Blackburn Trail Center (If you survive)." The tongue-in-cheek humor proved there was truth in advertising, at least in the wilderness.

Finally ascending to the hostel, I followed behind a retired priest who was slowly inching his way up the trail in obvious pain. "New boots, old age, and blisters, a deadly combination," he rasped. I offered to carry his backpack the rest of the way, but he mumbled something about offering his pain for Christ and needy souls. "Padre, some advice from an old altar boy. This isn't the Stations of the Cross, and we are not heading to Calvary," I chimed. He shook his head in frustration and allowed me to pass.

The Bears Den was a stone mansion, built in the 1930s by Dr. Huron Lawson and his wife, Francesca Kaspari, as a summer home. For hikers, it was a summer resort. For $25, I got a bunk with sheets and a pillow, laundry, a shower, a Tombstone pizza, a soda, and a pint of Ben & Jerry's. Free of charge was an exquisite sunset in the backyard at Bears Den Rocks, a rocky knob over 1,300 feet above the great expanse of the Shenandoah Valley. That evening in the bunkroom, the old padre was busy bandaging his feet. Needy souls would have to wait another day for redemption.

By morning, I was rested and ready to race the clock to Harper's Ferry. My goal was to reach the Appalachian Trail Conservancy (ATC) headquarters before closing time at 5 o'clock to register as a thru-hiker. At 4:10 p.m., I reached a trail sign that read

"Harper's Ferry 1.9 miles." I had fifty minutes to cover two miles of hilly terrain. The race was on! I started jogging when I crossed the bridge over the Shenandoah River and didn't stop until I reached the heart of the historic district. "Ah, shit," I yelled in frustrated disbelief as I looked around. I had missed the blue-blaze trail that led to the ATC office. I now had to walk up a steep hill for over half a mile. With sweat dripping off my face and my clothes soaked, I tapped on the center's door at 5:10 p.m. A staff member unlocked the door and hurriedly ushered me inside. I didn't beat the clock, but I won the race.

After gulping down a 32-ounce Gatorade, I had my picture taken in front of the building and registered as thru-hiker #386. With a huge sigh of relief, I trudged back down the hill. Wanting to get an early start the next morning, it was imperative to register today.

Back in the historic district, I stopped at the Outfitter at Harper's Ferry to visit Laura, owner and unofficial sutler for Herm's Hike. In 2008, Laura patiently talked and walked Brite and myself through everything that we would need, pointing out the pros and cons and answering our most trivial questions. Although it was a four-hour round trip from our home, it was time and money well spent. Until we put some AT miles on our boots, Laura had all the experience and expertise that we needed.

When it came time to purchase sleeping bags, Laura presented two Mountain Hardwear bags at $400 each. The price was dizzying, but this was top-of-the-line merchandise, and that's what I wanted. "It all compresses into this stuff sack," she said, holding up a minuscule nylon bag.

Calling her bluff, I proclaimed those immortal words that rolled off the lips of every hiker. "If you can fit that big bag into that little bag, then you just sold two sleeping bags," I joked in earnest. After a minute of furious stuffing, Laura handed me two small nylon sacks with a wide smile. In return, I handed her my credit card with a much tighter smile.

That evening I found a bed at the Town's Inn on the edge of the historic district. After dinner with fellow hikers across the street at the Secret Six Tavern (named in reference to John Brown and his conspirators), I returned to my room and anxiously waited for nightfall. Despite many visits to the national park, I had never explored the town under the cover of darkness. Excitedly, I stepped from the inn and walked into the pages of American history. With dim lights casting ghostly shadows against the buildings, it wasn't hard to picture the streets as they appeared during the 1860s. Any second I expected to see Union or Confederate soldiers marching down the street. Who knows, with a bit of supernal luck I might encounter John Brown himself. After peering into every storefront window and stalking the back alleys, I crossed the railroad bridge that spanned the Potomac River, retracing the steps of John Brown's raid. Heading back to the inn, I noticed a stiff breeze picking up from the southwest. Looking at the sky, wisps of dark clouds were crossing a vampire moon. Rain clouds were on the march. I just hoped the storm front was a day or two away.

The next morning, I was awakened by the sound of a pelting rain. Outside torrents of water rushed down the street. I checked with Karan the owner to see if I could stay another night, but the inn was booked. I had no choice but to hike.

Wearing a granny dress and sandals, Karan struck me as the stereotypical, older hippie chick. Noticing the religious trinkets and knickknacks scattered around her office, I commented on the Agape sign. "Unconditional love, that's a lesson you can learn on the trail. I've seen it in all shapes and sizes, kind of a variety pack," I intoned solemnly, hoping to delay my exit. My tactics worked. I had said the magic word: Agape.

For the next few minutes, we talked about my hike and her spiritual journey. Karan was a deeply religious person, active in her church and Bible study groups. Before I left, she asked if she could pray with me for a safe journey. As she placed her hand on my shoulder, I gazed despondently out the window. Upon finishing her prayer, I smiled weakly. I didn't know about her prayer, but my prayer definitely hadn't been answered. There were no last-minute cancellations on the rooms. I left the inn wondering where Karan was during the second week of August 1969, perhaps Max Yasgur's Farm. I wouldn't have been surprised to see her picture on the cover of the Woodstock album.

Crossing the bridge over the Potomac in the driving rain, I was finally in my home state. Any celebration was quickly tempered by the weather. Gale-force winds were whipping the river into a froth of brown, foamy water. The tide was running sideways with whitecaps crashing on the riverbank. With rain stinging my face, I hustled along the C&O Canal towpath for the next three miles. Entering the woods, I found relief from the wind but none from the rain. All day it rained in two modes, hard and harder.

As expected, the trail was deserted except for a group of teenagers and adult chaperones headed south. They were part of a Christian youth encounter group. From what I could see, they were not encountering a good time. Stretched out for over two miles, they lumbered past me in single file like a shipwrecked crew. I shouted words of encouragement over the wind and rain, but they only grunted or groaned in return. Many of the teens were hiking in blue jeans, tennis shoes, and plastic emergency ponchos. They were in dire need of an AT sutler like Laura.

I arrived at the Rocky Run Shelter feeling like I had fallen overboard. Everything was soaked. Even my Gore-Tex boots were soggy inside from the rain that trickled down my legs. My first order of business was to air out my hot, sweaty, and stinky feet. Since Damascus, my heels and toes had been peeling like an onion. It was a miracle that I didn't have trench foot. With only three hikers in a new shelter that slept sixteen, there was plenty of room to rig a clothesline for my rancid clothes and socks. The wet boots would have to wait for a sunny day.

By early morning, the rain had mercifully stopped. A blazing sun broke through the clouds and quickly dried the trail. Relishing the hot, rainless, windless day, I hiked twenty miles to Raven Rock Shelter for the night. The following morning, I hiked a leisurely five miles to Pen Mar County Park to rendezvous with Brite. When I arrived, she was on the road still two hours away.

To kill time, I visited the park's museum for an alluring history lesson. In 1877, the Western Maryland Railway opened an amusement park and resort at the site that quickly became a popular vacation destination. By the mid-1930s, the tourist boom went bust as Americans fell in love with the automobile and more distant vacation spots. The resort closed in 1943 and reopened in 1977 as a county park.

What piqued my interest at the museum was an old postcard on display. I immediately recognized one of the cards as the Buena Vista Hotel that once stood in nearby Blue Summit. I had been there as a child. With its towers, turrets, and wrap-around porch, the massive, three-story structure was impossible to forget. Catering to America's aristocracy, the hotel failed to survive the Great Depression and was sold to the Jesuits in 1931 for a retreat center. In 1960 and 1961, I had hiked to the hotel as a summer camper and peeked in the windows of this reportedly haunted mansion, my imagination running wild. In December 1967, the hotel, once the largest all-wood structure on the East coast, burned to the ground.

After my self-guided tour of museum and park, I still had an hour before Brite arrived. "It's only about a mile down the road. You can leave your backpack here," the attendant replied to my question about the location of Fort Ritchie. The postcard has sparked a road trip down memory lane.

I found my summer camp in a remote corner of the former army base that had trained linguists during WWII. Operated by the Baltimore City Police Boys Club, the camp director was my uncle John, my father's brother. Although the cluster of two-story, wooden barracks and the dining hall were long gone, I recognized the mountain lake where I first learned to swim.

Not only did I learn to swim, I learned gimp weaving, metal stipple art, archery, softball, kickball, and boxing. Staring through the fence, I remembered it all as if it were yesterday. Images of my youth floated across the empty field like rambunctious ghosts. I could see Officer John's ever-present smile and shouts of "Ah-choo, baby," his rapid-fire friendly greeting.

While headed back up hill savoring those sweet memories, a car pulled alongside with the windows rolled down. "Hey, marine, need a lift?" Brite shouted gleefully.

"Best offer I had all day," I replied, my smile growing wider. At the park, I retrieved my backpack and took some pictures next to the AT sign. After one thousand and fifty-four miles on the AT, I was finally homeward bound. I couldn't stop smiling. The trail had become a time machine with inflight beverages from the fountain of youth.

Chapter 15

A Father's Day Gift

(Parkton, MD, to Port Clinton, PA)

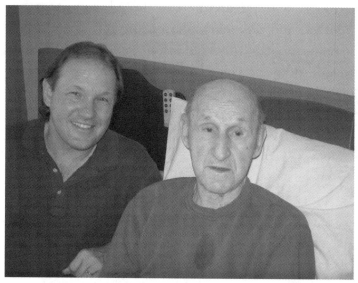

Father and son at the nursing home before the hike.

Before entering the nursing home, I took one last gulp of fresh air, fearful that I might suffer another anxiety attack like I did in Pearisburg. Nothing had changed in nearly three months. Most of the long-term-care patients were still living in suspended animation. Bob, my father's former roommate, was still walking the hallways around the clock on an unknown quest along an endless trail. I always wondered about his daily mileage. Surely, he had traversed the length of the AT since I've known him. I smiled at the thought of Bob with a backpack and hiking poles. I would have been honored to hike with him.

In my father's room, my mother sat by his side with other family members. Sitting in his geri-chair, the Buick of Alzheimer's patients, my father was holding court with a ceaseless barrage of babbling. We listened intently for a lucid comment, a gold nugget that could spark a memory and start a sensible conversation for a few seconds. We were desperately panning for Alzheimer's gold in a dry riverbed.

Once my father noticed me standing by his side, he immediately stopped talking. He slowly lifted his head and stared at me with a bemused smile as if trying to place an old friend.

"Hey, pal. Good to see you," he said warmly, extending his hand. Holding my hand firmly in his grip, he studied my face once again, tilting his head to the side for a better look.

"That's your son Paul," my mother remarked, pointing to my picture on the corkboard above his dresser. The board had become a pictorial family reunion that hovered over my father like a choir of guardian angels to remind him that he was not alone.

Twice my father shifted his gaze from me to the board, meticulously studying my photograph. "You know you're a pretty handsome fellow," my father proclaimed gleefully. Leaning toward my mother, he gently clasped her hand. "You know that man standing there looks a lot like me," he whispered loud enough to be heard by everyone in the room.

"He's your son," everyone shouted in unison. We laughed with tears in our eyes. My father looked at me and smiled. It didn't matter if he ever remembered my name again. The undeniable bond between father and son could not be erased. I was gone but not forgotten. I had found a gold nugget.

After everyone left for dinner, I stayed with my father to watch baseball on TV. As my father and I traded sporadic comments about the game, he reached out and placed his hand on top of mine. "That was close. He looked out to me," he blurted excitedly after a play at first base. With his eyes glazed by a milky film like a blind man, I wondered just how much of the world my father saw and understood.

Around the fifth inning, my father's hand slipped away. As he snored softly, I quietly tiptoed out of the room. On the door, I removed the red pin on the AT map that marked my progress and placed it in the center of the yellow dot that marked Baltimore. *Home is where you hang your hat, your heart, and your hike*, I thought. I left all three hanging in the room with my father. I would pick them up once the hike was over. Today there was no other place on the trail of life where I would rather be.

Back home after an emotionally exhausting day, I read the Father's Day cards from my daughters. With the oldest daughter in Alaska aboard a patrol boat and the youngest daughter performing in the great music halls of Italy with her college choir, I knew that a phone call was improbable. Gently caressing the cards, I traced my fingers delicately over the inscriptions as if reading braille, hoping to feel the love in the words. My daughters had affectionately referred to me as Sondance, but today there was no better trail name than Dad.

Vigorously and good-naturedly dissuaded by Brite about extending my stay, I hit the trail at Pen Mar Park after a two-day hiatus. Even though we were meeting in Duncannon at the end of the week, my adrenalin rush waned with each step. I was now walking away from home and my loved ones. There was no more lonely feeling. Like my father, I was heading in the wrong direction.

At around noon, I waded through a group of African American teenagers who were taking a break next to the trail. They looked at me as if I had just fallen out of the sky. "You're the first thru-hiker they've ever seen," piped one of the adult group leaders with Vision Quest. The kids were from the streets of DC and Philly, and this was their first wilderness experience. Last night they had camped in the woods and today they were hiking the AT. From the look on their faces, it was obvious they were not happy campers.

"Aren't you afraid they'll run away?" I asked the leader.

"Not a chance in the world," he chirped. "These kids are scared to step out of their tents, much less head off into the woods. This is the first time they've seen more trees than people. They're completely overwhelmed by nature."

As I headed down the trail, the counselor chased after me. "Could you do us a favor and talk to the group about your hike?" he pleaded politely. "Take this map and show them where we are and where you are headed," he added, handing me a trail map of Pennsylvania.

The teenagers were only mildly interested but totally flabbergasted that someone, especially my age, was walking from Georgia to Maine. "Why don't you take the bus?" one teen asked seriously. Lost for words, I blabbered about experiencing the last wilderness on the East coast. My comments fell on deaf ears. With three days left in their trip, they were already counting the hours before they could return to the land of concrete and convenience stores.

Continuing to hike, I pondered the lack of African American hikers on the AT. Since Georgia, I had met only a handful, three high school seniors on a graduation trip and two college students on a weekend trip with their fraternity brothers. The cost of equipment was often cited as the major obstacle to minority participation, but a good pair of hiking boots costs less than a pair of name-brand basketball sneakers. Sadly, the big athletic shoe companies are more devoted to perpetuating the pipe dream of a professional basketball and football career than promoting a healthy lifestyle in nature.

Inner-city kids like many of their white counterparts in the suburbs are suffering from Nature Deficit Disorder. They need to experience the joys, wonders, and health benefits of the great outdoors. But even if you give every child a free pair of hiking boots, there is another insurmountable problem. Greedily and gleefully, corporate America has spawned a generation of electronic junkies addicted to cell phones and video games. They have cleverly transformed the great outdoors into the great indoors.

In the early afternoon, I arrived at Caledonia State Park, a happy hunting ground for a hungry hiker. It was time to yogi. Sauntering through the picnic area, I spotted an easy mark, two young families at a shared picnic table.

"Where you headed?" one of the men asked.

"Maine," I replied, stepping slowly toward the table, pausing to wipe my brow for dramatic effect.

"Then you must be working up an appetite. We have some leftovers that we're throwing away. You're welcome to have it."

While entertaining my benefactors about life on the trail, I wolfed down two hot dogs, two hamburgers, two sodas, and a half a bag of potato chips. Before leaving, one of the moms handed me a twenty-dollar bill for Herm's Hike. To celebrate my good fortune, I stopped at the pool concession for an ice cream cone.

For the next two and a half miles uphill, I sweated and belched my way to Quarry Gap Shelter with the mother of all stomachaches. There I rested and digested in the shade by a spring-fed brook. With amenities that included hanging plants, reading material, and board games, the open log cabin should have been listed in *Better Homes and Gardens*. Instead of dinner that evening, I chatted with hikers that I hadn't seen since Waynesboro. Birch, Birdsong, Garage Man, and Pound Hound had hilarious tales about Mojo, who was reportedly still smoking his way to Mount Katahdin.

The following morning, I literally bumped into Sunnyside, the section ridge runner hired by the Potomac Appalachian Trail Club. I was heading north; he was heading south. We were both heading around a blind corner in a green tunnel. The affable young man was a roving goodwill trail ambassador who educated hikers about "leave no trace" ethics, performed light maintenance duties, and updated hikers on trail and weather conditions. For a young person with a love of the great outdoors, I couldn't imagine a better summer job. Even the chore of "knocking down the cones" at the privies was marginalized when compared to the other job perks.

I had spent two college summers in the sweltering heat at a plant that manufactured flame-treated, plastic containers. It was no wonder that I considered myself a "heat camel," someone who could walk for miles seemingly unaffected by the sweltering sun.

In the afternoon about two and a half miles from Pine Grove Furnace State Park, I officially passed the midpoint on the trail. Arriving at the park's general store, it was time to celebrate with another trail tradition. Feeling no effects from my previous day's eating binge, I dropped my backpack, boldly walked into the store, and purchased a half-gallon of chocolate chip cookie dough ice cream. The Half Gallon Challenge had begun.

I started slow and finished with a sprint, entering the record book with a time of 26 minutes and 16 seconds. With my hands raised triumphantly in the air and humming the theme from the movie *Rocky*, I reentered the store to claim my trophy, a small wooden ice cream spoon that said "Half Gallon Club." To date, the fastest time belonged to Fat Kid, who inhaled a half-gallon of ice cream in ten minutes flat. In a dairy stupor, that evening I rested comfortably at the Ironmaster's Mansion, more of a hiker's hotel than a hiker's hostel.

The next night I camped in the picturesque town of Boiling Springs. With no hostels, a trail angel family allowed hikers to pitch tents in their backyard for free. The other option was to spend a hundred dollars or more for a bed and breakfast. For penurious hikers, which included just about everybody, the decision was a no-brainer. For me, Auntie Agnes had become my all-expenses-paid vacation getaway.

The following morning, it was time to paint the town green. Inspired by the beauty of Children's Lake, a man-made, spring-fed, seven-acre lake, I stopped and retrieved the bag of Justin's poems from my backpack. For the next half an hour, I circled the lake and decorated the shade trees with poems. Children's Lake had unofficially become Poet's Walk. I just hoped the townspeople enjoyed the tree ornaments as much as I did.

Leaving town, I walked, not hiked, across the plains of Pennsylvania farmland. With no shade for the first ten miles, I melted under the scorching sun without a whimper. There were no rocks, ruts, or roots, and the heat worked wonders on old joints and muscles.

After a night at Cove Mountain Shelter, I hiked four miles to Duncannon. Since colonial times, the transportation hub had witnessed the passing of anything that moved on wheels or water, Conestoga wagons, ferryboats, Model-Ts, and steam locomotives. Bypassed by the interstate highway system, the town now served as a way station for AT hikers.

Downtown was an eclectic collection of old buildings with weathered sides and peeling paint. With its dusty and stained veneer, the gritty town had a charm that reminded me of Baltimore during my childhood. The streets were clean, homes were tidy, and residents were some of the friendliest people that I encountered on the trail.

My home for the night, the Doyle Hotel, was love at

first sight. Built in 1905 by beer magnate Adolphus Busch, the towering Victorian hotel was the last of the company's resort hotels. While the grand dame of Duncannon had survived over a century, she was now ostensibly showing her age that in many ways mirrored her tattered and tired guests from the trail.

For $25 a night, I got a bed with a pillow, a battered dresser missing half its knobs, a plastic chair, and a bare lightbulb overhead. For air conditioning, I simply propped open the screen-less window with a stick and hoped that I didn't fall out the fourth-floor window. The shared bath down the hall was musty and grimy, but the shower was hot and the toilets flushed. It was all a hiker could want. With its 1950s ambience, the rusty and dusty hotel would have been the perfect backdrop for a black-and-white movie like *On the Waterfront* or *Requiem for a Heavyweight.*

On the flipside, the one-star hotel featured a five-star tavern. Downstairs in the pub that evening, the atmosphere was friendly and lively with great grub and ice-cold beer. With its engaging owners Pat and Vicky behind the bar, the scene resembled the setting for the TV show *Cheers.* And just like the show, the owners and the regulars quickly knew your trail name.

The only opening for a seat was a barstool next to an attractive, nattily dressed woman. I didn't hesitate to grab it. While sipping our beers, we chatted about the hotel and the AT. Diane, who lived nearby, was waiting for her friend Bluebird, a thru-hiker from the class of '06.

"Stick around until she gets here. She'd love to meet you," Diane opined as she started to ask me about my hike. When I mentioned Herm's Hike, a pensive gaze suddenly veiled her face. "Let's find a table where we can talk with some privacy," she said, grabbing me gently by the arm and leading me away from the bar.

For the next half an hour, we talked with open hearts about our fathers. Both men were WWII veterans and career postal employees who were suffering from Alzheimer's. Their journeys from initial diagnosis to nursing home were nearly identical. The names Warren and Herman could have been interchangeable in their medical files.

"Paul, I'd like to help you any way I can if you'd like, maybe promoting the hike," she offered sincerely. Being a business analyst with a major health-care corporation in Harrisburg, she was an expert in marketing, public relations, and corporate communications. I readily accepted her offer.

When Bluebird finally arrived, the discussion shifted from fathers to hiking. To my delight, the effervescent and loquacious Bluebird was a wealth of knowledge about the trail ahead. In 2006 at the age of fifty-three, she suffered a hiker's worst nightmare. Two hundred miles before Mount Katahdin, she tore her rotator cuff and was forced to quit. Fighting a winter of depression, she rehabbed the shoulder after surgery and returned the next year to finish. Her hike like mine was a mission of mercy. Through the Hershey Company, her former employer, she had raised money for the Children's Miracle Network, a nonprofit that funded research, care, and treatment for sick children.

Her story got better with each passing minute. She had also written a book about her AT journey titled *Footpath My Ass*. I howled with laughter at the title. I had been repeating that mantra since Springer Mountain. No truer words had ever been spoken or written to describe AT.

On Saturday, after Brite arrived, I moved out of the Doyle and into a motel. We spent the day at the Billville Hiker Feed, a weekend of free food and events sponsored by Trail Angel Mary. On Monday, Brite went home and I went back to work. We would meet again in New Jersey.

Two days out of Duncannon, I caught up with Bookworm at the 501 Shelter, a fully enclosed bunkhouse with a solar shower. I had previously met him in Maryland. Today he was hawking trail magic. The prize package from another Mary, trail name Welsh Nomad, included slackpacking, a cookout, a night of camping in her backyard, and a brewery tour. Without hesitating, I readily volunteered to be one of the recipients.

The next morning, I hiked with Bookworm and four other happy hikers to meet Mary. About a quarter-mile from the rendezvous point on the mountain, the skies suddenly darkened and blotted out the sun. The air cooled drastically, raising goose bumps on my arms. Thunder boomed in the distance, growing louder with each step.

Minutes later, the wind roared through the woods with the deafening whoosh of a jet engine. In the blink of an eye, the feral storm was overhead with a cold rain that stung my face. Seconds later, jagged bolts of lightning stabbed the ground in violent explosions of white light that rattled my teeth. I was in a kill zone. Images of Albert Mountain flashed in my mind. I sprinted to catch Bookworm, not wanting to be the last man off the mountain.

"Hit the ground," Bookworm screamed as we came to a small clearing. With no escape route, I threw my aluminum poles to the side and dove head first into the muddy trail. The hair on the back of my neck bristled and tingled. Covering my ears with my hands, I lay motionless, waiting to be struck by lightning.

A minute later, the storm had passed and the sun reappeared. I retrieved my hiking poles and scraped the large globs of mud from my clothes. At the road crossing, Mary was waiting with snacks, beverages, and towels. With huge sighs of relief, hikers huddled in her van like it was a bomb shelter.

That evening at the cookout, Mary, a professional photographer, shared some of her latest photographs and her AT story. In 2004, in her late forties and feeling that life was passing her by, she decided to hike the trail. Battling hypothyroidism and fibromyalgia, she completed over seven hundred miles of the trail before succumbing to a knee injury. Although she never finished her hike, the experience had reenergized and refocused her life. She never needed to take another step on the AT. The trail had accomplished its mission.

The next day before hitting the trail, I sampled porters, ales, and lagers at the Yuengling Brewery in Pottsville, America's oldest brewery. Still giddy from escaping the electric chair, I overindulged and paid the price back on the trail. The first few miles uphill with a belly full of beer were agonizing, but I had no regrets. The beer had been cold and delicious.

Chapter 16
Rap, Rocks, and Rockamimi
(Port Clinton to Delaware Water Gap, PA)

Hiking out of Port Clinton, I had officially entered Rocksylvania, the land where rocks go to live and hiking boots go to die. The rocky terrain, which grew more ominous with each passing mile, was literally beating my feet to a bloody pulp. With my surgically repaired toes constantly twisting in my boots, my feet felt like they were on fire. Foot soaks and handfuls of ibuprofen, the only available treatment, became a daily ritual.

Coming into Palmerton three days later, I flailed and wailed along a path of jagged rocks as opposed to a rocky path. The trail had morphed into an industrial wasteland of discolored rocks, the byproduct of zinc mining. I thought I was hiking on Mars. From 1898 to 1980, the New Jersey Zinc Company, the largest producer of zinc in the United States, operated zinc mines and smelting operations. In addition to mountains of solid waste, the smelting process released toxic metals into the air and water that killed the mountain. Somehow the town of Palmerton had survived this industrial apocalypse and thrived. From the mountain ridge, it appeared like an oasis on the valley floor below.

That night I spent an enjoyable evening in the slammer. The town's old jail in the basement of City Hall had been converted into a free hostel. Somewhat dark and dank, the space had bunks, bathrooms, showers, and the right price. My cellmates were Gram Cracker and Rockamimi, two female hikers in their sixties whom I had met earlier.

The next morning the three of us climbed out of Lehigh Gap. For the eight-hundred-foot vertical ascent, I stowed my hiking poles in my backpack and climbed hand over hand to reach the top. On the ridgeline, the trail flattened out and offered stunning views of scarred and barren mountaintops. The size of the dead zone was staggering. Warning signs declaring the area a Superfund Clean-up Site updated the town's industrial legacy. On the lookout for rattlesnakes, we stepped gingerly over the rocks. No rattlesnakes were seen on the trail, but several were spotted in the prickly underbrush next to the trail.

Despite the punishing rocks, the miles melted away as Rockamimi and I swapped stories about our fathers. She had started her thru-hike in 2008 after her mother died. In June of that year, she left the trail after her father, a WWII pilot in the Royal Canadian Air Force, died from dementia. For two teary-eyed days, we opened our hearts to the healing powers of the trail. We agreed that there was no better place for grief therapy than the AT.

On the second day out of Palmerton with me lagging behind the speedy ladies, I stopped at PA 33 for a break. I was craving a bagel with cream cheese or an egg sandwich and a cup of fresh coffee. Just down the road, the town of Wind Gap had a Dunkin' Donuts and fast-food restaurants, but no public transportation. While standing by the road and deciding what to do, a tricked-out sedan with gold mag wheels stopped on the shoulder. The black driver with braided hair and gold chains was bouncing to the beat of the rap music blaring from the speakers.

"Man, you going to town. I'll give you a ride," he shouted out the passenger window.

"No thanks. I'm just resting here a little bit," I replied cautiously, not wanting to offend a trail angel. A quick ride into town would solve my food dilemma, but I wasn't sure if this was the right ride.

"What's your problem, man? You afraid that a black man is going to rob you and shoot you in the head?" the driver barked angrily, somewhat comically.

Shaken by his sudden outburst, I had to think fast on my feet before this uneasy encounter escalated into more than a difference of opinion. "No, man. It's not that. It's the music," I stammered, hoping to diffuse the situation with humor.

"I guess you want some of that redneck honky music like Willie Nelson."

"Yeah, that would be fine," I joked, hoping that would end the conversation.

"Shit! I knew it. Of all the people to help, I pick a country cracker," the driver fumed, comically shaking his head from side to side. After rifling through the glove compartment, he inserted another CD. Seconds later, Willie was joyfully singing about being "on the road again."

I shrieked with laughter. "I bet if I had long hair, you'd been playing the Grateful Dead."

"They didn't make the trip today. Now do you

want that ride or not?" he grinned, opening the door.

My trail angel was Glenny T., owner of Little City Music Recording Studios in nearby Brodheadsville and founder of the old school, soul, doo-wop, a cappella group 14 Karat Soul. Formed in 1975, the group had an extensive set of credentials that included *Sesame Street*, *Saturday Night Live*, Coca-Cola and Disney commercials, and opening for a number of big-name acts.

After returning to the trailhead with a bag of bagels lathered in cream cheese, we chatted for a few minutes about music and racial stereotypes. Glenny T. had escaped the ghetto in East Orange, New Jersey, to find inspiration in the Pocono Mountains. After telling him about my encounter with the Vision Quest hikers, we agreed that a mass exodus from the inner city to the mountains was long overdue. While I was impressed with Glenny T. and his music, he was equally impressed with my musical pedigree.

"You'll love this one," I boasted. "In high school, we had the Delfonics at our senior prom. After that, we went to a nightclub to see the Dells."

"Who would have thought that you're a soul brother? You've got to change your trail name from Sondance to Soul Dance," he chuckled before handing me his business card.

"Then you got to give me some soul, brother," I jived.

"What's your pleasure?" he crooned, his eyes flashing. Together we snapped our fingers and sang a couple of verses from "My Girl" by the Temptations. After that, Glenny T. disappeared down the road. Willie was still singing about being on the road.

Coming down the trail to the town of Delaware Water Gap, I fell hard on my right side after my foot became wedged in the rocks. Most of the impact was absorbed by my backpack. It had saved me again, but I was concerned about my recent balance problems. I had fallen in Pennsylvania more than any other time on the trail. Luckily, a nasty bruise was my last souvenir from Rocksylvania.

I arrived at the Presbyterian Church of the Mountain just as Gram Cracker and Rockamimi were leaving. They had finished their section hike and were going home. We hugged and said good-bye. Their camaraderie was going to be sorely missed.

The hostel in the basement of the church was a cozy clubhouse with bunks, bathrooms, and a communal space with comfortable lounge chairs. After a long, hot shower, I walked to downtown Delaware Water Gap, a quaint village nestled along the banks of the Delaware River. The only thing on my mind was food. I was ravenously hungry.

Although I had lost twenty-two pounds since Springer Mountain, my weight seemed to have stabilized. The old joke about "see food" was no joke. I was eating everything in sight. At the pizzeria, I had three slices of pizza. Working up an appetite, I walked over to the Apple Pie Bakery where I had the hot dog/apple pie special for $1.49. For dessert, I stopped at the convenience store for a pint of ice cream. Back at the hostel, I dined with a hiker named Star Trek, who prepared a gourmet burrito dinner from his mail drop. Feeling hunger pains later that evening, I walked back to town for more pizza and another pint of ice cream. That night, I drifted off to sleep with a full stomach, hoping not to dream of any rocks.

Chapter 17

Bears, Bugs, and Brite

(Delaware Water Gap to Unionville, NJ)

After a hearty and healthy (AT standards only) breakfast of two egg sandwiches, a bag of corn chips, a chocolate doughnut, a bottle of orange juice, and two cups of coffee, I threw the backpack against a sore shoulder and hiked across the Delaware River into New Jersey. Relief from the rocks was immediate. The I-80 bridge over the river was the longest section of flat terrain since crossing I-70 in Maryland. At the trailhead, Graham, a thirty-ish soccer coach from Nashville by way of Birmingham, England, was lacing up his hiking boots.

For the next six miles, we chatted about growing up in our native countries. A die-hard soccer fan, who had played at university and semipro level, Graham was slowly warming to American football and the Tennessee Titans. When the conversation shifted to must-see sights in the United States, I regaled him with stories of my travels out west. Like many foreigners, especially the Brits, he was enthralled with the legends of the Old West. By the time I finished my travelogue, he was ready to hike the Rockies, and I was ready to walk the Pilgrims Way in England.

While exploring the shoreline at Sunfish Pond, a forty-four-acre glacial lake, I was approached by Tim, a middle school teacher from New Jersey. He was scouring the area to interview a hiker for his next class. I readily agreed, honored to be a teaching point for today's youth. From his pack, he retrieved a small tape recorder and began the list of standard questions about hiking from Georgia to Maine. As for a final comment, I pasted together some quotes from Walt Whitman and a few of my trail thoughts. My message was short and sweet: "To find your true self, find your mountain. The trees will gladly and gloriously point the way. Take that hike into nature and let your soul stand cool and composed before a million universes." I thought it sounded pretty good and so did Tim. He gave me a donation for Herm's Hike with a satisfied smile.

While I talked, Graham walked. Once again, I was hiking alone. "Da bears! Da bears! Where are da bears?" I trolled merrily. With the highest density of black bears on the AT, I had yet to see any bear scat or tracks, much less a bear. A mile later, I turned a blind corner and came face to face with a large black bear.

It was mindlessly ambling straight toward me on a collision course. Startled, both of us froze in our tracks about ten yards apart. I instantly raised my hiking poles to make myself larger. "Run, bear, run," I yelled. The bear tilted his head and gazed at me as if to say, "What in the hell are you doing?" Remembering not to panic and run, I stood my ground and continued shouting. When I started to stomp my feet and wave my arms wildly, the bear turned on a dime and bolted into the woods.

When I finally reached the Appalachian Mountain

Club Mohican Center, a nature retreat for those seeking solace in the great outdoors, I was informed that a severe storm was forecast for late afternoon. Having gotten off to a late start due to my breakfast binge, I plunked down $25 for a night indoors with a bunk and a shower. As I was strategically selecting a bed close to the bathroom and far away from other guests, I bumped into Sue. An adult leader with Venturing Crew 125, an adventure program for male and female teenagers run by the Boy Scouts of America, she was preparing the group for an overnight hike on the AT. After a brief chat, I had a dinner invite.

Following a hearty meal of cheeseburgers and quesadillas, I repaid my gracious hostess by speaking about my hike. With a captive audience, I spent most of the evening answering questions about trail life and closed with my quote from Tim's interview. Afterward, Sue said that she would write about Herm's Hike on her blog. With two interviews under my belt, it was a good day to be a media star on the AT.

As I headed north the next day, I hiked a mountain ridgeline that provided a bird's-eye view of a valley that was dotted with lakes. Riding the thermals were jubilant shouts from summer campers that instantly triggered memories of Fort Ritchie. On a hot summer day like today, I would have sold my soul to be splashing in the water as a ten-year-old, even if it was a mountain lake at 8 o'clock in the morning.

Hours later, my summer daydream turned into nightmare at Brink Road Shelter. Since I was meeting Brite in Branchville the following day, I looked for a place that was close to the main road. I instantly knew this was not the place. I was standing in a drained swamp. The ground was spongy, and the musty, dilapidated shelter swarmed with huge clouds of gnats and mosquitoes. Several hikers had already set up their tents, but no one was venturing outside the safety of the insect netting.

With all the biting and buzzing, it was sheer insanity to stay. I pleaded with a handful of hikers loitering outside the shelter to follow me, but they were just waiting to set up their tents. I wasn't going to wait a second longer. Frantically I turned and sprinted back to the trail, swatting and fanning the black wave that followed me. The chase finally ended on the ridge when the swarm suddenly circled and headed back to the swamp.

Two miles up the trail, I found a small patch of thick grass on a bluff overlooking Lake Owassa and Branchville. Surrounded by light-blue clouds, dark-blue water, green trees, and gray rocks, I ate a quiet dinner and read a book in utter bliss until dusk. When night fell, I sat on a rocky perch and watched the light show below me that stretched to the horizon. Cars and trucks, homes and businesses, streetlights and traffic lights, all pulsated with a hypnotic, sonorous rhythm. Sitting on a mountain, I had never felt more safe and secure.

The next morning, I woke up early to watch a majestic sunrise. Although not the Smokies, being alone on any mountain was an inspiring way to start the day. While breaking camp, a group of bleary-eyed hikers stopped to take pictures. For them, it had been a sleepless night due to the relentless mosquitoes that slipped into their tents. From the look on their faces, I didn't have the heart to say, "I told you so." I hiked the remaining mile to US 206 giddy with anticipation. Brite was meeting me in Branchville.

On the highway, it was the Daytona 500. Rush-hour traffic was heavy, fast, and dangerous. Despite the endless parade of cars, I had no luck in hitching a ride. Reluctantly, I started to walk the four miles into town with my back to traffic and my thumb sticking out. Where was Slackpack with his friendly face when I needed him? After two miles of anguished walking on asphalt in the hot sun, a car pulled up behind me and honked.

"Hey, Sondance, get in! We'll give you a ride," the driver shouted. A wide smile creased my face. My trail angels were none other than Circuit Rider and Sherlock.

"Praise the Lord. I prayed for trail angels all morning and look who finally showed up," I exclaimed gleefully.

"We would have been here earlier, but you weren't too specific about the time and place in your prayer," Circuit Rider joked in reply.

"I'll be more detailed in my next prayer," I responded wryly, throwing my backpack into the backseat. Since I last saw them in Virginia, they had been jumping on and off the trail at various points to visit hiking friends and speak at local churches. Today, they were in town to visit Circuit Rider's mother. I was thankful that my trail angels had keen eyesight.

Brite found me napping on a bench in the borough's park square. After a quick hug and a peck on the lips, she staggered back as if she had been hit in the head.

"My God, you stink. You really reek to the heavens. You're not getting any closer until you take a shower and wash those clothes," she declared, waving her hand in front of her nose. Funny, but I didn't smell a thing.

After a weekend of day hiking and gourmet food, Brite dropped me off at the trailhead on Monday morning. It would be nearly two months before we'd meet in Monson, Maine. We calculated that if I averaged 15.5 miles a day with a zero day every seven days, I could get to Baxter State Park by mid-September. I was on target. Then again, I still had the hardest part of the hike ahead of me in New Hampshire and Maine. "Hey, Sondance, be careful out there. I love you," Brite shouted as I walked away. Oops, there was something in my eye again. For some reason, it happened every time we parted.

Chapter 18
The Brother and the Buddha
(Unionville to Kent, CT)

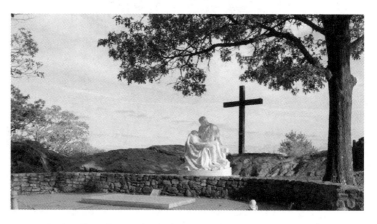

Father Paul's tomb atop the Holy Mountain at Graymoor.

Brite was heading for home and I was heading north, both of us eager to be heading out of New Jersey. Two days later, I crossed into New York. There was nothing special about the day until I crossed NY 17A late that afternoon. Like a mirage, the white silo of the Bellvale Farms Creamery glistened in the sun and beckoned. On a sweltering summer day, it was time for an ice cream break at the self-proclaimed best ice cream parlor in the country.

On this weekday afternoon, the place was

swarming with ice cream lovers as if all of New York were on vacation. After standing in line for about twenty minutes, I had my cone and found a seat at one of the crowded picnic tables. I licked away in ecstasy while enjoying a sweeping view of Warwick Valley from Mount Peter.

My appearance attracted the attention of some young children, probably no older than eight years, who began asking me questions about my hike. To them, I was a character right out of the Old West. They were flabbergasted when I told them that I, the Sondance Kid, had hiked from Georgia just to get an ice cream cone at the creamery.

"Mister, you must really like ice cream," a young, doe-eyed girl said in a whisper of a voice.

"No, hon, the Sondance Kid loves ice cream," I laughed, wiping ice cream from my face.

"Then maybe you should change your name to the Ice Cream Kid," she intoned with a serious look. I laughed even louder. My heart was melting faster than my ice cream.

Shouldering my backpack to leave, one of the parents asked me if I wanted another ice cream cone. I thought twice, remembering the Half-Gallon Challenge. Then again, I remembered never turn down trail magic.

The Ice Cream Kid walked back to the trail with ice cream cone in hand and a broad smile. Since reaching Virginia, ice cream had become a dietary staple to put some fat on my bones. Walking along the road, I could hear my father singing, "I scream. You scream. We all scream for ice cream," the refrain from the popular novelty song from the late 1920s. During those lean times, ice cream would have been a rare treat. Probably, that's why my father relished ice cream at the nursing home. He always attacked the bowl with childlike enthusiasm and a smile on his face.

My ice cream euphoria quickly melted in the heat. Getting to the shelter involved a number of hazardous rock climbs that required both hands. Once at the shelter, an even more dangerous scenario was unfolding. Two hikers were preparing to cook hot dogs for dinner. As the first drops of grease hit the flames, a huge black bear with a large white patch on its back appeared on the opposite ridge.

From our outpost above a wooded basin, we watched nervously as the bear moved closer before disappearing in the thick brush. After dinner, we stashed our food bags in the metal bear box, a sure sign of bear activity, and waited. Gathering as much wood as possible, we kept the fire going well into the night.

That night I slept along the back wall of the shelter in case the bear returned. Since I hadn't eaten any hot dogs, I hoped the bear would be smart enough to go after the dumb hikers who smelled like hot dogs. At breakfast, I noticed some large bear tracks in the mud about thirty feet from the shelter. On the trail, there were more tracks, possibly from a sow with cubs. Coney Island hot dogs belonged in a Coney Island stand not in an AT shelter.

The next day was a typical New York hiking adventure with frequent road crossings and a trail that bordered backyards. With no switchbacks, there were a number of nail-biting rock climbs that required patience, concentration, and balance. I thought that I had more than enough of the first two skills, but balance for a senior hiker was always marginal at best.

After scrambling up Agony Grind, a half-mile ascent on a five-hundred-foot rock pile, I nearly stepped off the side of Arden Mountain. Looking up for a white blaze and not looking down where I was stepping, I suddenly felt my foot drop as if I had missed a step on a stairway. There was no ground underneath me. My brain froze in terror. Instinctively, I grabbed a tree branch and swung back to the ledge like Tarzan. For a split second, I had lost my concentration and almost paid dearly for the mistake.

The geological highlight of the day was the Lemon Squeezer, an uphill alleyway between two rock walls. I twisted, turned, and pulled myself along with the palms of my hands. After stepping on air, there was nothing better than the feel of solid rock.

The William Brien Shelter, home for the night, was situated in a clearing just below a ridgeline. The squat stone shelter had bunks, a wooden floor, graffiti on the walls, and plenty of trash, the telltale signs of a road shelter. From the outside, the shelter looked like the perfect backdrop for a nativity scene. Just add some shepherds, the three Wise Men, and the Holy Family, and you had instant Christmas.

While I didn't have an instant Christmas, I had an early Christmas gift. Inside the shelter, I found an inflated heavy-duty rubber mattress and placed it under my tent. That night I slept on a ten-inch heavenly cloud of air. It was my most refreshing night of sleep on the trail. Little did I know that I would need it the following day, my most hectic day on the trail.

In the morning, I hiked the rocky ridgeline on

the back side of Bear Mountain to the Perkins Memorial Tower. The five-story stone tower, situated at 1,305 feet above the Hudson Valley, provided breathtaking 360-degree panoramic views. With interpretive signs, I easily spotted most of the nearby landmarks, but the Manhattan skyline to the east was hidden in the haze.

By mid-morning, Harriman State Park was reaching full capacity as people sought refuge from a summer in the city. In two hundred years, the only apparent change along the Hudson River was the size of the bank accounts belonging to the inhabitants. Once the exclusive summer playground of industrial barons, bankers, and bluebloods, the mountains and waterways were now the domain of the common picnicker.

Walking across the parking lot, a car slowly approached and stopped. Two white-haired ladies asked for directions to West Point and handed me a paper map. A paper map … I loved it. My kind of people!

After driving in circles, they were hopelessly lost. Having been at the military academy for business, pleasure, and a college recruiting trip with my oldest daughter, I knew the way. Before they left, there was one more question.

"Please don't be offended, but what's an older gentleman like you doing out here with that big backpack?" the driver asked.

"Bucket list item. Plus I'm trying to be a good son," I replied, taking a minute or two to explain Herm's Hike.

I anxiously watched the car exit the parking lot, hoping my directions had been understood. But instead of turning right to the main road, the vehicle turned left for another loop around the lot, stopping next to me. "How do you get lost in a parking lot?" I laughed aloud. They laughed with me.

"Here's a little something for your hike," the passenger said almost apologetically, handing me a crisp twenty-dollar bill. "My husband is in a nursing home with Alzheimer's. God bless you, Sondance. You'll be in our prayers." The day was off to a great start.

Crossing underneath the highway, I walked the trail on the winding asphalt path through the Bear Mountain. At 124 feet above sea level, it was the lowest point on the AT. As planned at the start of the hike, I stopped at the Walt Whitman statue for a moment of reflection. One of my literary uncles with Emerson and Thoreau, Uncle Walt had been calling me since high school.

In "Song of Myself," he invited me to explore my spirituality. In "Song of the Open Road," he invited me to hike the AT with these words: "Afoot and light-hearted, I take to the open road, healthy, free, the world before me, the long brown path before me, leading wherever I choose."

Gazing up at the nearly nine-foot statue, I easily pictured Uncle Walt on the trail, trail name Leaf for his iconic literary work *Leaves of Grass*. With his long beard, flowing hair, and floppy hat in hand, all he needed was a backpack to start chasing the white blazes. "Thank you for the invite. Glad that I could make it," I whispered, hoping not to attract the attention of visitors.

Exiting the zoo, I started the walk across Bear Mountain Bridge. Built in 1924 and measuring nearly a half-mile long, it was for a time the longest suspension bridge in the world. Today it was the longest section of flat trail on the AT. As I stepped on the span, two hikers stopped in the middle, waved, and waited. It was Circuit Rider and Sherlock.

"We thought we saw you in the park. When I looked behind and saw the blue headband, I knew it was you," Circuit Rider intoned. "How are you since New Jersey?"

"Rev, I'm worried that I might be running out of gas," I declared dramatically. "I'm constantly hungry and I've been falling quite a bit recently."

"Maybe you need to take some time off. We're heading into Peekskill for a few days. You're more than welcome to join us," he suggested with a concerned look.

"No thanks. Have to keep moving. Maybe I'll take a few days rest at the next good hostel." The generous offer was tempting, but I wanted to keep moving. Like other hikers, I had become addicted to mileage. It was a bad habit that was hard to break.

"In that case, let's pray for your health," Circuit Rider declared with a nod from Sherlock. Bowing our heads, we joined hands one hundred and fifty feet above the water. Suspended between heaven and earth, there was no finer church. As Circuit Rider called on the Great Physician to give me strength, I was certain that boats passing underneath thought we were leaping to our deaths in a bizarre hiker's ritual. In reality, it was only another leap of faith.

"I hope to meet you guys in the Whites when I'll need my prayer prescription refilled. I'll be easy to spot," I joked as we reached the other side and parted company. Unknowingly my blue headband had become my signature trademark.

Late that afternoon, I arrived at the Holy Mountain, home of the Graymoor Spiritual Center and the Franciscan Friars of Atonement. Picking up a self-guided tour brochure at the gift shop, I began exploring the grounds. Atop the seven-hundred-foot summit of Mount Atonement was the Holy Spirit Chapel with stained-glass windows featuring Saint Claire and Saint Francis. Within a few steps of the chapel was Calvary Rock, the tomb of Father Paul, a former Episcopal priest who founded the order in 1899. On a rock outcropping overlooking the grave was a replica of Michelangelo's Pieta in front of a towering white cross.

While sitting on a bench next to the statue and enjoying the view, I was approached by a maintenance worker who had been cutting grass. I feared that I was going to be evicted for a breach of religious protocol, such as snacking at Father Paul's tomb.

"We don't get many hikers on the mountain. Just wanted to make sure that you weren't lost and looking for the campground," he said politely.

"No, nothing like that. I'm just an old altar boy enjoying the tour," I replied, waving my brochure.

"Do you have some time for the real tour?" he asked.

"The rest of the day. I'm staying at the campground tonight," I answered, wondering what was the real tour.

"Wait right here while I find your tour guide," he replied before hurrying back to the chapel.

A few minutes later, he returned with an older gentleman dressed in work clothes similar to his. "I'm Brother Pius, gardener, historian, librarian, and man about the mountain," the man said with a warm smile and firm handshake. "Jimmy, here, said that you like history."

"Big-time history buff. Nothing better than the history of old churches," I replied emphatically.

"Well, then follow me. I'll give you the grand tour that won't cost you a dime." I followed Brother Pius to his car.

For the next two hours, we visited every historic and religious site in the area. Brother Pius was an encyclopedia on the history of Graymoor. Born on a farm in Cape Breton Island, Nova Scotia, he traded the corporate world and his girlfriend for life as a friar after attending a weekend religious retreat. He arrived at Graymoor in 1955. His pastoral assignments included ministries in England before returning. Now he worked at keeping busy in retirement. At least we had one thing in common.

I told him about growing up Polish Catholic and attending a Catholic high school run by the Franciscan Friars. I sealed a bond of friendship when I told him about my aunts, Sister Regina and Sister Loretta. He marveled at the ministry of Sister Loretta, who at eighty years of age was walking the streets of Trenton, New Jersey, and administering the sacraments to the elderly and infirmed. "Now you know where you get your hiking genes," he kidded.

My tour included the 9/11 prayer garden that featured a cross made with steel beams and rebar from the World Trade Center, the abandoned foundation that was to be the national shrine to Saint Anthony, and a chapel that housed the small shed where Father Paul lived for a year when he first arrived at Graymoor.

The highlight of the tour was the chapel of Saint Francis of Assisi, a miniature cathedral with a vaulted ceiling, wooden beams, stained-glass windows, and facing high-back pews. The altar once stood on the site where Saint Francis received his stigmata (the wounds of Christ). Looming over the altar was a statue of Saint Francis. The contemplative face was molded from one of the two known death masks of Saint Francis. It was so life-like that I expected the patron saint of ecology to climb down and join us. Before leaving, Brother Pius asked if I would like to pray with him. As he prayed, I looked up and wondered how Francis would have prayed with us. It was then that I realized that Francis was standing before me in the persona of Brother Pius. Following Brother Pius out of the silent sanctuary, I mentally noted that my prayer bank had received the day's third infusion of spiritual currency. Being a trail yogi now had a new meaning. Instead of soliciting picnic baskets, I was gathering prayers in a holy almsgiving. Back at the parking lot behind the main building, Brother Pius had one more question.

"What's the one thing you miss most on the trail?" he asked with a mischievous grin.

"My family," I responded immediately.

"No, I meant something to eat. You mentioned that you were always hungry."

"Bread and butter," I blurted. "Make that fresh bread."

"Follow me," he ordered as he led the way to the main building. Disappearing into the kitchen, he returned with a bag of rolls in one hand and a Styrofoam container in the other. Back at Father Paul's bench, I dined on a feast of roast beef, mashed potatoes, and green beans with a generous supply of rolls and butter squares, well out of sight of my fellow hikers.

After a busy day of meeting and greeting, I looked forward to a good night's sleep. As I walked across the ball field to the campground and pavilion in the shadow of Holy Mountain, a man was waving his hands in the air and shouting.

"Who wants to get high with me? I got grass and booze," the man yelled repeatedly at the top of his lungs while a boom box blasted heavy-metal music. On top of a picnic table was a half-gallon of whiskey, a case of beer, and a couple bags of grass. Two other hikers in the pavilion were somehow going about their business, ignoring the bellicose and obnoxious intruder. Mustard, who claimed to be a thru-hiker, had been at the pavilion since noon. However, no one ever remembered seeing him on the trail.

At dusk, three more hikers arrived, one of them a college librarian named Karen. She had planned to section hike in Maine, but the swollen rivers had changed her plans. Tall and attractive with a long blonde ponytail, she immediately attracted the romantic interest of Mustard. After an hour of pestering questions and lewd comments, Karen had enough.

"No wonder your wife left you. You're a disgusting, drunken bum. No woman in her right mind would want to sleep with such a pathetic excuse for a man," Karen shouted in his face. "And turn off the music. We're here to sleep." I took an instant liking to the woman.

"Hey, I just wanted someone to party with," Mustard muttered before turning off the music.

With this uneasy truce, I grabbed my backpack

and pitched my tent in the field. The only sounds for the rest of the evening were the hourly bells from the chapel tower. I slowly drifted to a peaceful slumber, replaying the day's events.

My father would have been thrilled to meet Brother Pius since Saint Francis and the Franciscan Sisters of Saint Joseph were his religious heroes. As for myself, my hero of the day was Brother Pius. He, like my two Franciscan aunts, truly lived the words of Saint Francis: "We have been called to heal wounds, to unite what has fallen apart, and to bring home those who have lost their way." If there was a Catholic Hall of Fame, all three should be enshrined.

The next morning there was no sign of Mustard after his verbal castration. I never saw or heard of him again. At one time, Graymoor allowed hikers to sleep in the dormitory section of the main building. Mustard was living proof why that policy was discontinued.

At around noon, I crossed NY 301 with Beach Boys music playing in my head because I was headed to the beach. "Surf's up," I shouted merrily to the trees. About a mile east of the trail was Clarence Fahnestock State Park that featured a lake and a concession stand. Once I saw water, I threw off my backpack and hit the beach running. The first thing I lost was the hiking boots. Walking on sand was the perfect massage for my battered feet. The next thing I lost was my shirt. Diving into the cool water for a mountain baptism was physically and emotionally rejuvenating.

After lounging in the sun, I headed to the concession stand. While wolfing down a couple of hot dogs, I struck up a conversation with a retired couple on a day trip. After telling them about my day at Graymoor, they looked at each other and grinned.

"What do you think about the Buddhists?" the lady asked politely.

"I love the Buddhists. You know the sacred mountains, prayer wheels, prayer flags, the Dali Lama, the art of compassion," I replied, not knowing what they had in mind.

"We're headed to a Buddhist monastery just down the road. You're more than welcome to tag along."

"Are you Buddhists?" I asked.

"More like Zen Catholics," the lady answered as they both laughed.

The offer was enticing, but I thought long and hard. In southern Appalachia, just down the road or just around the bend could be twenty or thirty miles on a one-lane country road.

"How far down the road?" I asked. "I'm kind of pressed for time."

"A couple of miles. We'll bring you back."

The deal was sealed. My hosts Phil and Barbara, both retired schoolteachers, frequently visited the monastery and Graymoor to worship. By embracing Buddhist dharma (dogma) and meditation, they discovered a deeper appreciation of their birth faith.

"Enlightenment and eternal life are goals on our spiritual journey. Saint Francis and Buddha are kindred spirits in many ways. So why not borrow from the best," Phil philosophized. There was no argument from me.

Like Graymoor, I found the Chuang Yen (meaning "majestically adorned") to be exhilarating. The path leading to the main temple was lined with statues representing disciples of Buddha. I easily pictured Brother Pius and my aunts joining the ranks. Inside the Great Hall, I stood spellbound at the sight of Buddha Vairocana. At thirty-seven feet in height, the statue was the largest indoor Buddha in the Western Hemisphere. Just as amazing was the Lotus Terrace, a horseshoe-shaped tier of ten thousand smaller statues of the Buddha that surrounded the giant Buddha like fans at a stadium.

Outside the manicured grounds included more statues, more shrines, and a koi lake. Done in the architectural style of China's Ming Dynasty, the buildings resembled the Shaolin Monastery in China, referenced in the TV show *King Fu*.

Like Graymoor, there was a palpable stillness in the air that awakened the senses. I walked slowly behind Phil and Barb in harmony with my surroundings. That afternoon, the monastery had become an extension of the AT and another shelter from the storm of everyday life.

Back at the trailhead, I thanked my gracious hosts for the enlightening experience. With palms together at my chest and hands pointed upward, I bowed to my trail angels. "Namaste," I whispered reverently, recognizing the divine spark in my trail angels. They returned the greeting with angelic smiles.

That evening, I met up with my hiking group at RPH Shelter, a cinder-block garage with a covered porch and delivery service. Over a pizza dinner, I replayed my day at the beach and the monastery.

"In two days, I've met three of my heroes, Walt Whitman, Saint Francis, and the Buddha, all giants in the compassion hall of fame. These guys are definitely at the top of my dinner list with the dead," I joked.

"What about Jesus Christ? I'm sure you met him at Graymoor. No room for him at your banquet table?" a Bible-toting hiker interjected sarcastically, obviously not sharing my religious diversity.

"I've already dined with him. You know, Holy Communion," I replied curtly. The cluster of hikers laughed heartily.

The next night at Telephone Pioneers Shelter while drifting off to sleep, I noticed a sweet fragrance in the air, a rarity in the shelters. I had noticed the scent lingering in the air at rest stops and figured it was just wildflowers. Rolling over in my sleeping bag, my faced brushed against something silky soft and flowery sweet. Opening my eyes in the dim light, I saw it was Karen's long hair. Somehow she managed to wash her hair every evening on the trail. In my stupor, I was tempted to gently caress her hair in my fingers and press it to my cheek. However, sanity prevailed when I realized that I might be hiking to Katahdin with my arm in a cast.

The next day I crossed the railroad tracks at the Appalachian Trail station, nothing more than a wooden platform with yellow handrails, a blue bench, and a bulletin board. A couple of hikers were already waiting for the metro to New York City and a sightseeing vacation. Later in the day, I crossed Hoyt Road and entered Connecticut. The "deli run," as New York was known, was over. With only fifty-two miles of the AT, Connecticut ranked just above Maryland as the shortest state. Three days later, I hiked with Karen into the town of Kent as the sweet fragrance of flowers lingered in the air. All I could hear was Scott McKenzie singing his 1967 hit, "San Francisco (Be Sure to Wear Flowers in Your Hair)." All I could picture was Karen with the flower children and the Summer of Love when peace and love reigned supreme.

"Karen, if you're going to San Francisco, be sure to wear some flowers in your hair," I crooned as we walked. Karen just smiled and winked. Flower Power lived!

Chapter 19

You Can't in Kent, or Can You?

(Kent to Glen Brook Shelter, MA)

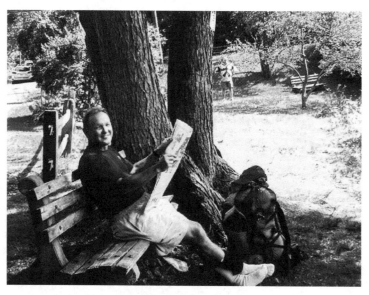

Home is where you hang your hat and drop your pack. The bench was my bed for the night in West Cornwall.

On the way into town, we passed through the campus of the Kent School, a private, co-educational college preparatory school that resembled an Ivy League college with its stately brick buildings and tree-lined walks. Like the Kent School, the town of Kent was trendy, preppy, and expensive. Hikers weren't openly welcomed but tolerated within reason. Hikers often joked that Kent should change its name to "Can't."

After a frustrating search, Karen found her car in a shopping center lot and headed home. I reluctantly said good-bye and quickly headed down the main drag to find the hiker essentials, a pizza parlor, a laundromat, and a bank. But all I really needed at the moment was money and a place to stay. There was free camping behind a house on the main street, but with the weather forecast calling for heavy thunderstorms, I was looking for a bed indoors.

With thunder booming in the distance, I hurried over to the ATM outside the Bank of America. After inserting my credit card and entering my codes, the screen reported that my withdrawal of $200 was complete. The screen was flashing green, and I was seeing red because I never saw the cash. Sensing a scam, I ran into the bank a minute before the front door was locked.

"Travers was my maiden name," the teller chuckled as she examined my driver's license. "If you don't mind me asking, what's your nationality?"

"My mother is Polish and my father might be German and English. He's not really sure because his father died when he was an infant," I replied.

"Well, this is your lucky day, the luck of the Irish, you might say. Your last name is Irish. I traced my ancestry back to a village in Antrim County in the early 1600s."

"Now I know why I have a fondness for Guinness and Irish whiskey," I joked as she handed me my cash.

"By any chance are you Polish Catholic?"

When I answered yes, she then asked me if I had heard of the Shrine of Divine Mercy in nearby Stockbridge. Although I had never been there, I told her that I was familiar with the place from my aunt Sister Loretta.

"Paul, you need to visit there. You are on a pilgrimage, and I believe it's part of your journey," she implored.

Shortly after the death of her husband, Geralyn prayed at the shrine during a devotion to Saint Faustina, the Polish nun who founded the Divine Mercy, a devotion to the merciful love of God to be shared with those in need. On Divine Mercy Sunday, while looking at the sky, she experienced a radiant light that washed away her overwhelming grief.

"As a matter of fact, I'm carrying a Sister Faustina prayer card, a traveling gift from my aunt," I replied, retrieving the card from my backpack.

"It's like you're an answer to my prayers," she replied softly, her eyes tearing. The words of Cee Cee echoed in my mind.

Back on the street, it started to rain. At the campground, the lawn was already a wet sponge. My only option was a local bed and breakfast. After a number of calls, I found a room at the Cooper Creek B&B, three miles north of town. Fifteen minutes later, Mary, co-owner with her husband, Cooper, whisked me away to a soft bed and a hot shower. With rain pelting the car and the windshield wipers swinging furiously, I realized that I had found the best bargain in Kent. By now, the campground was under water. Arriving at the yellow clapboard farmhouse that dated to the 1830s, I found my connection to Emerson and Thoreau. With uneven wide-plank pine floors, warped glass in the windows, and fireplaces in nearly every room, the house was iconic New England.

The next day with the rain still falling, I took a zero day to do laundry. With the laundromat deserted and no one on the streets, I discreetly removed all of my clothes and lounged in my Gore-Tex jacket that extended to mid-thigh. About an hour later, I discreetly slipped on warm, dry pants and a t-shirt. Not a soul had entered the building. A few years later, I learned that hikers had been banned from the establishment for indecent exposure. While I'm sure I wasn't the first hiker to launder au natural, I proudly took credit for the ban to ensure a place in trail lore.

The following morning, I walked the trail along the Housatonic River under sunny skies. The miles were easy and the mosquitoes immense. To avoid being eaten alive by lunchtime, I lathered my face, arms, and legs in a thin layer of deet. The bugs didn't stop buzzing, but they did stop biting.

Deciding to treat myself on this lazy summer day, I hitched a ride to Baird's General Store at the junction to Cornwall Bridge. "Best subs in New England," the driver proclaimed cheerfully, handing me a five-dollar bill in the parking lot. "Buy yourself lunch or give it to your hike."

Baird's was an old-fashioned general store, circa early 1900s, with a deli that didn't disappoint. My Italian cold-cut sub was as good as advertised. On the front porch, I dined with Steve, a local resident. Every Sunday morning, he stopped at Baird's to eat and dispense advice to any wayward and wandering hikers.

"Don't let Kent fool you. It just likes to appear haughty. The villages heading north are just as friendly as the ones down south. It's just more reserved and refined. After all, you are in New England," he scoffed in a fake English accent with an emphasis on the word "new." After finishing our meals, he gave me a ride back to the trailhead and a $10 donation for Herm's Hike.

Back on the trail, I was in a hurry. The owner at Baird's, who was working behind the deli counter, had been watching the final round of the British Open on TV. Tom Watson at nearly sixty years old was attempting to become the oldest golfer to win a major championship. Since turning fifty, I rooted for the underdog and the over-the-hill, no matter what the sport. With a five-hour time difference, my only hope of watching any more golf was a play-off. That was enough incentive to hike faster.

At the road crossing to West Cornwall, I quickly hitched another ride to the village. Inside the Smokin' BBQ, I spotted the owner of Baird's at the bar watching golf. He invited me to join him for a few cold beers on his tab. To our disappointment, Tom lost in a four-hole playoff. At the end, Tom just ran out of gas. I knew the feeling.

After wolfing down a bbq sandwich, it was time to explore the village. Walking down to the river, I found a grassy area with a couple of park benches near the iconic red, covered bridge that spanned the Housatonic River. Following my custom for park benches, I sat down and enjoyed the parade of people. In the river, a flotilla of kayakers and canoeists dodged fishermen and wading children. Above the river, painters were attempting to capture the idyllic beauty of a summer Sunday afternoon.

Dozing off under rapture of the scene, I decided the bench would be my home for the night.

When the crowd had thinned, I retraced my steps through the village in search of more food. Crossing the railroad tracks, I entered the Wish House, a gift and clothing boutique. With the few stores already closed, this was my last chance for ice cream.

"Hello! Anyone home?" I called out, slowly walking to the counter. The only sound was the creaking of the floor. The store was deserted. In the back of my mind, I heard Rod Serling from the TV show *The Twilight Zone* introducing tonight's episode: "Paul Travers, known as Sondance, the Sondance Kid or simply The Kid, is a man wishing to solve the mystery of life by venturing into the wilderness on the Appalachian Trail. But he needs to be careful where he searches. He is moving into a land of shadow and substance, of trees and mountains, of people and places. Today he has entered the house of his wishes in … the Twilight Zone."

Suddenly, there were light footsteps behind me. I quickly turned, my backpack hitting something hard with a metallic clang. Pirouetting like a ballerina, I caught the swaying card rack with my hand. Spinning back around, I was now face to face with Bianca, the store's owner.

"Just looking for a birthday card," I stuttered embarrassingly.

"Nice footwork and great reflexes," she joked cordially. "If you need help, just let me know. We don't get too many hikers in town. We're a little off the trodden path."

I bought a birthday card for my oldest daughter, and then I stayed to chat. After telling Bianca about meeting noted labor historian, author, activist, and filmmaker Jeremy Brecher on the trail earlier in the day, she confirmed my suspicion that Cornwall was home to the rich and famous due to its proximity to New York. In addition to Henry Kissinger in Kent, area residents included Paul Fusco (creator of *Alf*), Michael J. Fox, Michael Palin, Jane Curtain, and Whoopi Goldberg to name a few. Meryl Streep lived up the road in Salisbury.

After mailing my card at the post office, I headed back to the Smokin' BBQ where I was invited by Mike and Lisa to join them for dinner. They had seen my backpack and were curious. For the next hour, I regaled them with tales from the trail. When it came time to leave, my hosts graciously picked up the tab for another BBQ sandwich and gave me $20 for Herm's Hike. I was beginning to lose count of how many free meals and how much money I received that day.

Back at the park bench, I enjoyed a fiery orange sunset that faded to embers of muted red and purple behind the mountains like a Van Gogh painting. The student painters should have stayed longer. In the cool of the evening with the parking lot empty, I dug out my sleeping pad and sleeping bag and placed them on the bench. Like Glasgow without the rain, I was tramping and feeling the freedom of the open road. It was exhilarating.

Just as I finished making my bed, a bright light suddenly swept the area. Fearing it was the police, I crouched behind the bench and held my breath. A car door opened. *Just my luck! I'm going to be arrested for trespassing in a deserted park. I just hope the bunk is soft*, I thought, stifling a laugh.

"Sondance, are you there? It's Mike from the

restaurant."

Recognizing the voice, I jumped to my feet. "I thought you were the law," I laughed aloud madly.

"Thought you might like a late-night snack. A little AT room service," he chuckled while handing me a pan-size pizza.

After my late-night snack, I climbed into the sleeping bag. Closing my eyes, the bubbling and gurgling river sang a soothing lullaby. With people popping in and out at a moment's notice, the day had been like a surreal dream. Their generosity was humbling. Steve at the deli had been right about New England.

The next morning before sunrise, I walked across the covered bridge and hitched a ride to the trailhead in a pickup truck full of construction workers. About five miles down the trail, I descended the ridgeline and walked to Falls Village. The mosquitoes welcomed me back to the Housatonic River. Taking a break at the power plant to apply deet, I struck up a conversation with a local resident who was taking an early morning stroll. When the conversation turned to my father's battle with Alzheimer's, the woman started to cry and clenched me impetuously in a bear hug.

"Last year my father committed suicide by placing a bag over his head after he was diagnosed with the disease," she said sadly, stepping back and wiping away the tears.

"I'm so sorry," I said in a faltering voice. I reached out and gave her a hug, my shirt wet with her tears.

For the rest of the day, I was lost in my thoughts about Ann and her father. When there was no cure for a horrific disease, was suicide selfless or selfish, courageous or cowardice? I had no answer, only the final question that my mother always asked: Why does God let bad things happen to good people? That's what religions have been trying to answer since the dawn of mankind. Following a skillfully crafted script, they attempt to humanize and rationalize the mystery with a cast of characters and stories. Satan, original sin, free will, divine plan, redemptive suffering, heavenly reward, eternal damnation, reincarnation, or natural order, no one really knows. All you can do is embrace the mystery. Pick one, some, none, or all for comfort and wait for the real answer when your mortal clock has expired.

Too much time to think and no scenery to drink, I thought. My brain was more tired than my legs. I needed to energize my spirit and clear my mind. Finally at Rand's View, I found that "awe" moment. As if stepping through a magical door, the trail opened to a lush green mountain meadow that funneled into a green valley. In the background, waves of green mountains rolled to the horizon under an ice-blue sky. I had no doubt that today God's favorite color was green.

"Thank you, God! Thank you, God!" I shouted at the top of my lungs. I threw down my backpack and danced a jig. Dropping to the soft grass, I propped my head against the pack and soaked in the scenery, letting the sun caress my face and melt away my worries and cares. I could have easily spent a relaxing night in the meadow, but the day was still young.

About half a mile from the road to Salisbury, I spotted three hikers meandering up the trail. The first hiker to greet me was an older gentleman in hiking clothes who looked to be in his eighties.

"You don't mind if I hold you up, young man? The Mrs. isn't doing too well, but still likes to hike," the man said politely. The first to arrive was an older lady, obviously the gentleman's wife, quickly followed by a middle-aged woman who was the couple's daughter. As we chatted, I noticed that the older lady was unusually quiet and stared constantly at the ground. I recognized the symptoms immediately.

"My mom has Alzheimer's, but getting outdoors seems to lift her spirits. So I try to get both of them out whenever I can," the daughter said.

"From a good son to a good daughter, good luck on your journey," I said to the woman after telling her about Herm.

Walking down the gentle hillside, I thought about my father in the great outdoors as an Alzheimer's patient and shook my head in frustration. On both occasions, we read from the same script. "Where are you taking me? Are we going home?" my father would repeat nervously as I pushed his wheelchair out to the patio.

"No, Dad, not home but outside to sit and talk. You need a change of scenery," I would reassure him. Outside, he became quickly agitated, clearly unsettled by his new surroundings.

"Hey, mister, why are you doing this for me? Do I owe you money?" he would inquire with a confused look.

"It's because I love you," I would chuckle, hoping to ease his fear.

"Boy, that's really something," he would respond with an impish smile. After a few minutes, he would fall soundly asleep, and I'd wheel him back to his room.

My father's comfort zone, his world, was limited

to the second floor of the nursing home. Anyplace else was unexplored wilderness. I often wondered if any research had studied the beneficial effects of nature on Alzheimer's patients. Maybe the best therapy was to have all nursing homes with Alzheimer's patients adjacent to nature preserves.

Outside the food market in Salisbury, hikers were feasting on ice cream. I quickly bought a pint and joined them. Two hikers, whom I hadn't seen since Hot Springs, commented about my weight loss, saying I looked like a prisoner of war. And if I was looking to spend the night, there was space at Maria's. They had canceled their reservation to attend a music festival.

Before heading to Maria's house just a few blocks away, I stopped at a couple of churches, the town library, and the Salisbury Historical Society to drum up business for Herm's Hike. After my face-to-face encounters with Alzheimer's earlier in the day, I felt compelled to make the extra effort regardless of how tired I was feeling.

I found Maria sitting in the shade on her backyard porch. Taking a seat, I noticed the sign hanging on the lattice wall that said, "Maria Loves Hikers." I took an instant liking to her. She was caring, charming, sassy, and witty, a lot like my mother.

Being the only guest that night, I dined with Maria and her son. Afterward we spent the evening on the porch talking, or I should say Maria talked and I listened.

Originally from the Dolomites, Italy's northern Alps, she was abandoned by her mother as a young child and adopted by a farming family. Until she married a GI at the end of WWII, she tended dairy cows, a task she equated with slave labor. As a teenager under Nazi occupation, she had buried a small suitcase with her treasured possessions, a few pictures, some letters, and some jewelry, under a chicken coop so Hitler wouldn't steal them. She wondered if anybody had ever discovered her treasure chest, hoping that someday it could be returned to its owner. Once in America, she and her husband settled in Connecticut, living in a farmhouse with no heat or plumbing. Not that much different from her home in the Dolomites, she concluded, but she had her freedom.

The next morning I was out of the door before Maria appeared. I opted not to eat breakfast, breaking one of Maria's house rules that a hiker never leaves hungry. With the sun shining, I was hoping to push a twenty-mile day and finish near Great Barrington. After a three-mile climb from Salisbury, I enjoyed a dazzling view of western Connecticut from Lion's Head before heading to Brassie Brook Shelter for a break.

"We should try to get him to the road. That way they won't have to waste time backtracking," I overheard one hiker declare nervously outside the shelter.

Peering inside the shelter, I saw the reason for concern. An older hiker in his fifties or sixties, whom I had seen about a week ago, was propped against the wall in his sleeping bag mumbling incoherently. A hiker was at his side, coaxing him to take a drink from a water bottle. Although rescue units were on their way up the mountain, a few of the gathered hikers felt a sense of urgency.

"What do you think?" one of the hikers asked me, once again probably equating my age with wisdom or experience in these matters. Luckily, I had a little of both.

"What did 911 say?" I asked.

"They said keep him warm, awake, and hydrated."

"Then that's what we should do. Look, these people are trained for this kind of work. Let them do their job," I replied. My logic prevailed, and each of us took turns watching over the patient. In the meantime, I rifled through the hiker's backpack for some ID to give to the authorities. Luckily, I found his wallet stashed in a plastic bag inside one of the pockets. I also searched for any medicines or prescriptions, thinking his condition might be health related. About an hour later, the rescue unit arrived. After taking vital signs, they placed the hiker on a litter and hooked up an IV bag. An ambulance was waiting at the bottom of the mountain. Suffering from an apparent mental breakdown, the hiker had remained in the shelter for three days with no food or water.

Chapter 20
Arlo's, not Alice's, Restaurant

(Glen Brook Shelter to North Adams, MA)

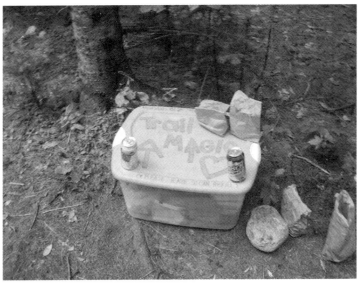

Trail magic in any fashion was always celebrated with giddiness. Like finding an extra present under the Christmans tree.

That evening at Glen Brook Shelter, the conversation was about the old man. I noticed that every time the subject of older hikers surfaced, furtive glances were cast my way. Just because I looked older didn't mean I wasn't young at heart. After all, I had grown old without growing up, or at least that's what a lot of people said. But age did have its advantages on the trail. I could relate to things that were impossible for them, and one of those things was waiting for me tomorrow. If I was a pilgrim from the '60s, it was time for a pilgrimage to the shrine of the '60s that included a free lunch.

The next morning after an eight-mile downhill hike to the US 7, I quickly hitched a ride into Great Barrington.

"Where you headed?" the woman asked.

"Trinity Church," I replied excitedly.

"Arlo's place. I know exactly where it is," she chirped. Sliding in the front passenger seat, I held my backpack in my lap. Every inch of space was crammed with clothes, books, and household items. Christa was in the process of moving from Long Island to the Berkshires. Her new mountain home was going to be her salvation.

A professional landscape designer to the rich and famous in the Hamptons, she was starting a new life in her forties after battling addictions to booze, drugs, men, and money. Sober for over seven years, she had found a God of second chances who was now directing her life through the power of prayer. In the parking lot of the Guthrie Center, she handed me a postcard for her book *Silent Screams from the Hamptons*, a memoir about overcoming the "silent screams" of everyday struggles. She apologized for not finding a copy in all the clutter.

A few steps later, I was standing at ground zero for the '60s. The Guthrie Center, formerly the Trinity Church, was one of the great hippie landmarks of the '60s; in my mind second only to Max Yasgur's farm, the site of the 1969 Woodstock concert. In 1965, the Gothic structure with its distinctive bell tower, then the home of Alice and

Ray Brock, became immortalized in hippie folklore. After Thanksgiving dinner, Arlo Guthrie, folksinger and son of legendary troubadour Woody Guthrie, and a friend offered to take out the trash. It was a trash talk that transformed a life and defined a culture.

Finding the local landfill closed, the men tossed the garbage down a ravine where other rubbish had been previously dumped. Both men were later arrested and convicted of littering. As a result of his criminal record, Arlo was rejected for the military draft, or so the story goes. His Thanksgiving misadventure spawned a hit record *Alice's Restaurant Massacree* and a hit movie *Alice's Restaurant.*

Inside the building, now a community center and performing arts venue that also hosted interfaith worship services, the walls were adorned with pictures and posters of Woody, Arlo, and other artists. Above the hallway was a sign that read "One God — Many Forms / One River — Many Streams / One People — Many Faces / One Mother — Many Children. Ma."

Ma was Ma Jaya Sati Bhagavati, a spiritual master who taught that divinity manifested itself in many ways beyond words and form. Her interfaith doctrine embraced the belief that all paths of love led to the truth. Ma's mantra was my latest spiritual epiphany. It was the essence of human spirituality. There was no such thing as one true religion or one path to salvation. God created diversity; man created conformity. If I was God, I would revel in the diverse expressions of divine worship. To say only one prayer or sing only one song in one tongue would be blasphemy. Imagine a world with only one kind of tree, flower, or animal. Imagine a world with only one kind or color of people. I imagined John Lennon should have written another verse about nature in his song "Imagine."

While browsing the musical memorabilia, I met George, the director of the center and good friends with Arlo. I asked him about Arlo's whereabouts and mentioned my invite to Rising Son Records, Arlo's record label. George only commented that Arlo stopped by once in a while. Understandably, he didn't want to divulge information about his boss to a stranger who could be a celebrity stalker.

My invite to the record label came the previous year after I had contacted a handful of celebrities to promote Herm's Hike. I asked only for a quote to post on my website. Donations were never mentioned. I wrote to First Lady Nancy Reagan, Olympic gold medalist Dorothy Hamill, sportscaster Jim Nantz, and Arlo. All were connected to the Alzheimer's Association except Arlo. He made my list because he lived near the trail and his family had experienced the nightmare of Huntington's disease. Maybe he would be a sympathetic soul and offer a few kind words for publicity.

My only response was from Mrs. Reagan's press secretary, who politely declined. With Arlo, I was more persistent. After a couple of e-mails to his record company, I received a reply thanking me for my query and inviting me to stop by if I was in the area. I knew I was being blown off, but an invite is an invite. My only problem was how to get from the trail to the record company, which also happened to be Arlo's home.

Before leaving, George invited me to stay for lunch. I graciously accepted and was led to a table where a number of senior citizens were seated.

Today the center was the Guthrie Bistro. Lunch was made from scratch with fresh ingredients. The menu included a salad, meatballs, a vegetable, bread, dessert, and beverages. While talking with my fellow diners, I couldn't stop smiling. Here I was in the great room of one of the most hallowed sites in pop culture enjoying a gourmet meal.

"I heard you talking to George. I think I might be able to help you get to Arlo's place," the man next to me said. Leaning over, he whispered details about a cryptic road. "Takes you down to his driveway, but don't tell him I sent you," he laughed.

Back on the trail, I headed to the East Mountain Retreat Center for the night. Once again crossing the Housatonic River, I spent the next eight miles fanning insects from my face. The interfaith center was the perfect way to bookend the day after my visit at the Guthrie Center. Secluded in the woods, the center was a sanctuary for people to reflect, heal, meditate, and explore their spirituality. With quiet hours, a silence rule, and a bedroom for snorers, it was also the perfect place for a good night's sleep.

While lounging in the dayroom, a ghost from the AT appeared in the doorway and pointed at me. "I met you and your wife at the Hiawassee Inn," the man beamed. Just Tim, a retired Special Forces soldier and AT veteran, had been driving the shuttle van.

"You look a little thinner since the last time I saw you. You need to keep eating to keep up your strength," he chided. There was that weight issue again. The next morning as I was heading out, he gave me his collapsible mosquito hat. "You're going to need this more than me, at least until you get to the Whites," he said, sympathetic to my complaint about the insects.

After spending the night at Goose Pond Cabin, once a private summer retreat that had been converted to a comfortable hostel, I headed out with the first group of hikers. While crossing over I-90, I stopped in the middle of the bridge and waved my hiking poles above my head, honoring my AT tradition. I always wondered how many drivers looked up and wished they could trade places with me if only for an hour. "Look at that guy up there. He's free. Free to roam the countryside. Free to come and go as he pleases," they would hopefully say. Within seconds, my presence was acknowledged with the blast of an air horn from a tractor-trailer. Long-distance drivers like long-distance hikers knew the freedom of the open road.

A couple hundred yards beyond the bridge, my hike almost abruptly ended. While crossing a wooden footbridge, I slipped and fell flat on my back, nearly toppling into the creek. While wiping the globs of green, slimy moss from my clothes, I cursed my inattention. Any wet wood is dangerous, regardless if it's a bridge or a branch. Once again, my backpack took the brunt of the painful blow. For the rest of the day, I slowed my pace to avoid the wet rocks, moving like a man in a minefield.

At mid-afternoon, I arrived at the blueberry farm, home of the famous Cookie Lady. No one was home and there was not a cookie in sight. Retrieving my map and companion book, I plotted my course of action. I was about seven miles from the next shelter and ten miles from Dalton, the nearest town. Somewhere nearby was the mystery road that led to Arlo's place.

Leaving the farm, I promptly came to a decrepit,

unmarked dirt road that headed east. I wasn't sure if this was the road described by my lunch partner because it wasn't hidden, although it was mysterious. Throwing caution to the wind and the rain, I turned right and followed the old road. As predicted, it eventually dead-ended into a gravel road. Not sure where I was, I turned right again and walked downhill, the easiest option. After passing a few houses, none that looked like an office for a record company, I hit a two-lane paved road.

"Two rights do make a wrong," I wryly lamented. I trudged back up the hill to see where a left turn would take me. I immediately spotted a sign that said "Hippie Road." I was on the right road.

Minutes later, I was standing in front of a sprawling farmhouse. Behind me was a white nondescript building that resembled an oversized garage. I waited for a few minutes, hoping that someone would notice my presence. Taking a deep breath, I started for the front door of the house when I heard a door open behind me.

"Rising Son Records?" I asked the lady who was heading to her car.

"Through the door," she answered.

Hearing voices inside, I gently knocked. "It's open. Come on in."

"I didn't hear from Mr. Guthrie, but I received this invite," I stammered, explaining Herm's Hike while pulling out a copy of the e-mail. The four ladies seated around a table looked at one another with amused grins.

"We don't get too many walk-ins, especially with backpacks," said one of the ladies, whom I recognized as Annie Hays Guthrie. Annie, Arlo's middle daughter, was the head of the record company and an outstanding folksinger in her own right.

"Since I walked over fifteen hundred miles to get here, do you think I could meet your dad and get a picture for my trail journal?" I added nervously, knowing this was my moment of truth.

"He's home but not home at the moment, away on business. But you can meet and take a picture with us," Annie chuckled.

For the next thirty minutes, I chatted with the staff, had a cup of coffee, and took a few pictures with Arlo's daughters. Before leaving, Annie gave me two of Arlo's CDs. Outside in a steady rain, I walked back to the dirt road, disappointed that I didn't meet Arlo but glad that I had met part of the family. That alone was a good story for my trail journal.

It was a shame that Arlo and I didn't meet because we were kindred souls. Arlo's spiritual journey had taken him from his Jewish heritage, to the Franciscan monks, to the Buddhists, and finally to a Hindu guru. His road to enlightenment had come full circle from the back door of the Trinity Church to the front door of the Guthrie Center. Through Ma, he embraced all religions as "different views of the same reality." My spiritual journey was still a work in progress with the belief that all religions were different paths to the same mountain. *One Mountain – Many Paths and Many Prayers*, I thought. Ma would have approved.

Leaving the office in late afternoon, I needed to eat. Taking Annie's advice, I hitched a ride to two cheeseburgers and fries at the Becket Country Store. After my meal, a considerate customer, taking pity on a wayward hiker, gave me a ride back to Arlo's driveway.

Walking back uphill in a blinding rain, night was falling fast. I now needed a place to sleep, and that's when the idea hit me. "The band bus. The perfect shelter," I said to myself. If the boys from the Greasy Creek Friendly could sleep in abandoned cars then I could sleep in an abandoned bus.

Under the cover of darkness, I tiptoed back to the record office. There was a new band bus parked next to the building, but I didn't want to be arrested for breaking and entering. Instead, I opted for the junkyard in the backyard where two derelict buses were parked in the weeds. Crouching low to avoid the lights from the house, I circled behind the one closest to the tree line. I was in luck. The door was slightly ajar. I opened it just enough to squeeze in sideways without my pack. Adjusting my eyes to the darkness, I found a cushioned bench and unrolled my sleeping bag.

Warm and dry with raindrops pinging the bus, I closed my eyes and imagined the songs and stories that had been swapped in this very bus. A million miles and a million smiles, the bus had a memory of its own. Maybe that's why Arlo kept the old buses around. They were part of his life's story and had become family heirlooms.

Somewhere in the distance, a freight train sounded its horn. I hadn't heard that lonesome sigh since my night in Glasgow. It always made me think of home and my loved ones so far away. As I drifted off to sleep, the sound of Arlo singing "Hobo's Lullaby," one of Woody's songs, played in my head like a scratchy record on an old phonograph. "Hey, go to sleep, you weary hobo. Hey, let the towns go drifting by. Hey, can't you hear the steel rail humming? Well, that's a hobo's lullaby." There really wasn't too much difference between life on the rail and life on the trail.

I hurriedly packed and left the bus before sunrise under clear skies. By daybreak, I had retraced my steps on the dirt road and was back on the trail for an easy ten-mile hike to Dalton. At around noon, I crossed the railroad tracks at the edge of town and walked down the street to the home of Tom Levardi. It was hard not to miss the two hiking poles stuck in the front lawn.

Tom was New England's answer to Bob Peoples. He generously opened his home to hikers, providing a place to sleep, shuttle service, and ice cream sundaes. All he asked in return was that hikers remove their shoes before entering the house.

That afternoon, I headed into town to promote the hike. My first and only stop was the Dalton Methodist Church just up the street where the sidewalk in front of the church was the AT. The office was closed, but I heard music coming from the worship area. Standing in the rear, I watched the contemporary music group rehearse. When the band took a break, Meg, the lead vocalist, waved me over.

"How can we help you?" she inquired warmly.

"I'm hoping you could mention my hike in your church bulletin or newsletter," I replied, handing her a Herm's Hike flyer.

"Why the churches?"

"Because my hike has become a spiritual journey," I replied, mentioning my various prayer encounters.

"Would you like to speak tomorrow at our Sunday service?" she immediately asked. Without hesitation I accepted, not sure what I was getting into. I had walked the walk, now it was time to talk the talk. "Ask for Lisa tomorrow before the service. I'll let her know that you're coming."

The next morning, I was called to the front of the congregation after a scripture reading. For the next ten minutes, I spoke emotionally about my family's battle with Alzheimer's, my spiritual journey, and my prayer encounters on my hike.

"How did you find our church?" one lady asked at the coffee and cake social after the service.

"I don't think I found your church. I think my trail angels did. I just followed them to the front door," I chuckled.

As I said good-bye, Lisa handed me a packet of scripture readings and prayers for hope, healing, and salvation. She said that my appearance had been more than a fortuitous coincidence. Both of Meg's parents had battled Alzheimer's.

After draining the last of the coffee and stuffing my backpack with the last of the doughnuts, I exchanged contact info with Lisa and stepped on the trail for a pleasant Sunday stroll through the woods. About a mile and a half from the town of Cheshire, I followed a marble trail that led to the Cobbles, a scenic overlook with stunning views of the Hoosic River valley and the menacing Mount Greylock in front of my face. Tomorrow's destination was proof that I was back in the big mountains.

Since it was Sunday, it only seemed natural that my home for the evening was Saint Mary of the Assumption Church. Inside the parish hall that served as the hostel, I tossed my backpack onto a couch in one of the side rooms. In the kitchen, I found a small, battered, well-worn transistor radio with a broken antenna that miraculously worked. After dinner, I stretched out on the couch, ready for some music.

Deftly manipulating the station dial, I struck gold. The Who were singing "Summertime Blues" on Casey Kasem's American Top 40 radio program for the week of July 25, 1970. For the next two hours, Casey counted down the hits with songs from Three Dog Night, Elvis, CSN&Y, James Brown, Bread, and Stevie Wonder. I was floating on a cloud of sweet memories from that summer. I was eighteen years old, officially retired from baseball, had raised my GPA to avoid flunking out of college, found a summer job at a plastics factory, and fallen in love. I wasn't singing the blues that summer.

Later that night, my moonlight serenade with Casey ended abruptly when four hikers burst through the front doors like a bomb. Talking and laughing loudly, they entered my room and started to take off their backpacks. Wet and muddy, they looked as if they had been dragged up and over the mountain.

"Holy Jesus, you guys stink to the high heavens. If you want to sleep here, you going to have to clean up," I admonished as the stench of raw sewage burned my nose. Looking up, I noticed the small red scabs. "What in the hell happened to your faces?"

"Black flies," they shouted in unison. Without another word, they filed out of the room to find another space.

The next morning I lathered up in deet and pocketed my net hat for easy access. The hike to the summit was an invigorating eight miles with an elevation gain of 2,500 feet. As I hiked higher on a gorgeous summer day, the air grew cooler and the bugs disappeared. As I headed up, my thoughts tumbled down to the church in Dalton.

My talk about the power of prayer had been well received, but I wondered if I should have spoken more freely from the heart. Over the past four months, my concept of prayer had changed. With mankind's history of death and destruction, much of it due to religious ideology, I was no longer certain if God answered prayers or even bothered listening. I did know for certain that we could be the answer to prayers, either ours or someone else's. That belief in the power of compassion and unconditional love was enough to change my concept of prayer.

For me, prayer was no longer a petition but a conversation that connected me to God's divine love that was the DNA of our souls. Having that divine spark, we could connect with anyone and anything in the universe. When we transmitted our love to others through prayer, our communal souls vibrated at an ultra-high frequency in unison. That's when miracles happened. And if you prayed because it felt good or connected you to God in some other manner, mission and miracle accomplished. *Many paths to the mountain – many prayers on the mountain*, I thought, unconsciously channeling Ma.

After lunch on the mountaintop at the Bascom Lodge, I joined the swarm of day-trippers who were enjoying the stunning views. At 3,491 feet, Mount Greylock was the tallest mountain in the state and the tallest on the trail since central Virginia.

In July 1844, Thoreau hiked to the summit and spent the night in a wooden observation tower. Some literary scholars believed that Greylock was the mountain baptism that led to his grand experiment in simplicity and self-efficiency at Walden Pond. It wasn't difficult to comprehend his wilderness rebirth where I stood.

I walked the paths and searched for the stones that had memorable quotes from Thoreau. I finally found my favorite one hidden by the branches of a spruce tree, actually hidden by nature. Uncle Hank would have appreciated the irony. It read: "It were as well to be educated in the shadow of a mountain as in a more classic shade. Some will remember, no doubt, not only that they went to college, but that they went to the mountain." Too bad Thoreau wasn't around in 1969 as a college professor. I would have been the first in line to sign up for the class that no doubt would have included a field trip on the AT. Fast-forward forty years later as a student of life, I was finally walking in the footsteps of Uncle Hank, trail name Walden. I wondered if I was now eligible for a Thoreau wilderness scholarship for seniors, not students but citizens.

On the recommendation from Just Tim, who had given me his personal list of hiker friends and hostels, I spent the night at a local hotel that was heavily discounted. With a Mexican restaurant, a pizza parlor, and supermarket across the street, it was the ideal location to refuel for the day and resupply for the week ahead. That evening just before sunset, a brilliant double rainbow appeared over the mountains to the north. I saw it as a good omen and phoned Brite with the good news. Rainbows and a hiker named Rainbow Brite were synonymous with good luck. I only wished that I had a fortune cookie to confirm it.

Chapter 21

Sunset on Sondance

(North Adams to Rutland, VT)

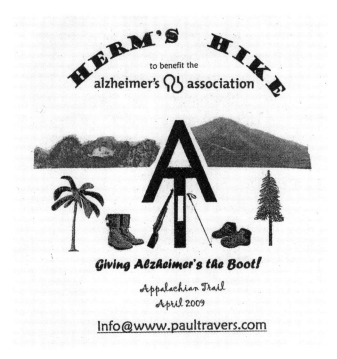

Herm's Hike poster with Bloody Nose Ridge and Mount Katahdin in background.

The next morning, I crossed the Hoosic River and followed the white blazes through a backyard into the woods. Four miles later, I entered Vermont and chalked up another state, but there was no cause for celebration.

Once in Vermont, you were immediately reminded and reprimanded that you've done 80% of the miles but only 20% of the work. Hard to believe the next three states were the toughest, but it was true. For the next 105 miles the AT followed Long Trail, the oldest and one of the most rugged long-distance trails in the country. The state itself was jokingly called "Vermud" by hikers. With one of the wettest summers in history, the endless supply of mud was thicker than maple syrup.

My hike to the summit of Glastenbury Mountain, the first mountain in Vermont, was short and steep. On the wooded peak, I climbed the fire tower high above a forest of red spruce, balsam, fir, and hemlock. At the top, it was easy to see how someone could be devoured by the wilderness. The view was an endless, undulating, thick carpet of green that looked the same. Walk fifty feet off the trail, turn around, and you're lost forever. Any call of nature needed to be heeded very close to the trail.

Back on the ground, I listened to a hiker expound on the region's history. "Locals call these woods the Bennington Triangle, our own version of the Bermuda Triangle. Since the late '40s, people just disappear like they walked off the face of the earth. Strange lights and sounds, UFO and Big Foot sightings," he extolled dramatically. I took note when he said that two of the missing were named Paul and Paula.

At Stratton Mountain, the birthplace of the AT, I paused for another history lesson. According to the bronze plaque next to the tower, Benton McKaye, father of the AT, was sitting in a tree atop the mountain when he was inspired to create the AT.

After a night at the Stratton Pond Shelter, I

hitched a ride to the outfitters in Manchester Center to resupply and refuel. The sales assistant said the boutique town was a draw for celebrities throughout the year. Last year, Sylvester Stallone, Rocky Balboa from one of my all-time favorite movies *Rocky*, had picked up a hiker. I hurried to hitch a ride back to the trailhead. "Yo, Paulie, need a ride? Hop in," I could hear Rock say.

Three miles up the trail, I found myself at the summit of the Bromley Mountain Ski Resort. In almost every direction, ribbons of cleared forest ran down the mountains. This was the heart of Vermont ski country that attracted skiers from around the world.

With the ski lift closed for the day, I decided to join the other hikers and cowboy camp on the mountain. After three nights in a shelter, a night under the stars would be a special treat as long as it didn't rain.

At around 1 a.m., I crawled out of my sleeping bag to enjoy the celestial extravaganza and walked quietly to the edge of the summit. Everyone was sound asleep. Staring once again at the stars, I revisited my experience on Max Patch Bald in similar dramatic fashion. Focusing on stars directly overhead, I wondered what light was my soul in the vast expanse of an endless universe. I sat down and stretched my arms to the sky, closed my eyes, and tilted my head backward. Seconds later, I felt my body floating above the mountain, pulsating with a radiant energy toward a star that burned brighter than the others. I was headed for my star. Time had stopped; the world below ceased to exist. My earthly link had been broken. I drifted to the edge of the cosmos like a vaporous cloud, translucent and transient, before dissolving into deep and dark velvet sky. Feeling the wind against my face, I opened my eyes and landed softly back on the mountain.

Back in my sleeping bag, I stared at the stars until they were indelibly etched in my memory. I wondered if death was simply the soul drifting through the universe to reconnect with the Creator. In my head, Don McLean sang a gentle lullaby: "Starry, starry night, Paint your palette blue and gray, Look out on a summer's day, With eyes that know the darkness in my soul." Tonight God the Artist had provided the palette; Don the artist had painted the words.

Three days out of Bromley, I climbed the rocky side trail to Killington Peak, the second highest peak in Vermont at 4,235 feet. On a clear day, you can see the White Mountains. Today I saw only mountain silhouettes in the hazy sunlight. After lunch at the summit restaurant, I hiked down the mountain to US 4 where I hitched a ride into Rutland.

Home for the night was the hostel at Back Home Again Café. Since Springer Mountain, I had heard some outlandish and opinionated stories about its owners, the Twelve Tribes of Israel. Now it was time for Paul the Pilgrim to determine if the religious group was a cult, the occult, or a credible cultural covenant with God.

Started in 1972 as a coffee shop ministry for teenagers by Gene and Marsha Spriggs, the group was labeled a cult by local religious leaders and run out of town. They ran from Chattanooga, Tennessee, to the mountains in Vermont. Blending Christian fundamentalism and Messianic Judaism, they believed the Messiah would return when the first-century church with a New Israel, consisting of Twelve Tribes in twelve locations, was restored.

After a free beverage, I was escorted upstairs where there were bunkrooms for each sex, bathrooms for each sex, and a common area with a kitchen. Literature about the group, which made for interesting reading, was readily available.

Like any religious movement, they openly recruited. I could see where their cafes, bakeries, stores, and farms would be selling points. Broken people, searching for a spiritual home, could easily be attracted to their communal lifestyle and sense of family. All you had to do was give up your material possessions, take a Hebrew name, and follow the teachings in the Old and New Testaments.

In my "good book," compassion was the foundation for any valid religion, and they seemed to have it. From the outside, they weren't ostensibly a cult. To me, their only fault was their austere interpretation of the Bible. Then again, selective interpretation seemed to be the subjective foundation of every book religion.

After breakfast the next morning, I made a donation and boarded the shuttle that operated between Rutland and Killington. While castigated for their religious beliefs, they couldn't be criticized for their culinary talents. The food and the service were amazing. If they ran their church like their café, maybe in a few hundred years or so, they might be considered a mainstream religion. Stranger things have happened in the religious realm.

Minutes later, I was dropped off on a lonely stretch of highway surrounded by mountains. With cool temperatures and overcast skies, it promised to be a perfect hiking day.

A few miles down the trail, I walked through

Gifford Woods State Park and chatted with some of the park staff. After passing Mountains Meadow Lodge next to Kent Pond, I headed toward Thundering Brook Falls where I planned to take a break.

Heading down the wide, well-maintained trail, I increased my stride. Suddenly I was violently slammed to the ground from behind. "Ahhh," I screamed as I landed on my right shoulder with a stabbing pain. Lying on the ground, I looked up to see who had pushed me. There was no one. Looking behind me, I saw a tree stub, a common hazard on newly cut trails, no more than two inches in height protruding from the ground.

"Son of a bitch, bitch, bitch," I yelled in pain and frustration. I released the straps on the backpack and slowly rose to my feet, my right arm hanging limply by my side. "Can you believe this shit?" I shouted angrily, walking in small circles while gently massaging my shoulder. With any movement of my arm, the pain only increased. Having had surgery on both shoulders for torn labrums, I knew the white-hot pain of a serious injury.

Taking deep breaths, I stood grim-faced and considered my options. I could walk uphill to the park office or walk down to the road just ahead. I grabbed my backpack in my left hand and limped to the road. To make matters worse, my right knee was also hurting.

Other than a painful shoulder and knee, I had some bloody scrapes on my right forearm and right knee where I landed. Breaking open my first aid kit, I was cleaning dirt from my wounds when a car slowly approached and stopped.

"Are you okay?" the driver asked after rolling down the passenger window.

"I think I just busted up my shoulder falling down this hill. I can't move it," I said in obvious pain with a greasy sweat beading on my face. Don got out of his car and walked over for a look.

"Jesus, you looked like you just got done wrestling a bear," he joked, trying to ease my pain. "Can I do anything for you?"

"Do you think you could take me to a hospital or clinic in town?" I groaned grimly.

"No problem. I'm just out running errands." Don helped me into the car and threw my pack into the backseat. Underway, he asked me about my hike. When I mentioned Herm's Hike, he suddenly stopped talking. "I lost my wife a couple of years ago to Alzheimer's," he stuttered weakly.

Fifteen minutes later, Don led me through the doors of the medical center in Rutland. Before leaving, he gave me his phone number. "If you need anything, and I mean anything like a ride or a place to stay, just call me. Hey, us old guys have to stick together," he reassured.

X-rays revealed no broken or fractured bones. That was the only good news. The grim diagnosis was a sprained shoulder, or in medical terms, a Type 1 shoulder separation that involved a partial tear to the acromioclavicular (AC) ligament or other ligaments that connected the collarbone to the shoulder blade. Treatment was ice to reduce pain and swelling, a sling until the pain subsided, and over-the-counter pain and anti-inflammatory medications. The knee fared much better with a diagnosis of Grade 1 sprain with swelling and stiffness. Treatment was RICE: rest, ice, compression, and elevation.

"How long before I can get back on the trail?" I asked the doctor nervously.

"Depends on how quickly you heal. Could be anywhere from a couple of weeks to a couple of months. But with your history of shoulder problems, you should have an MRI to determine if there's any other soft tissue damage," he replied.

For the first time since I fell, it dawned on me that my hike might be finished. Since turning fifty, it took me twice as long to heal from an injury. Even though the last operation on my right foot was over a year ago, it often felt like I was walking on pebbles. It didn't hurt; it just didn't feel normal.

At the Comfort Inn down the street from the hospital, I immediately began treatment with ice and ibuprofen. That evening I called Brite with the latest update. I said that it was a slight shoulder sprain that needed a few days of rest. I didn't mention the knee. With Brite being a former orthopedic nurse, I knew she wasn't buying my story.

After three days of lounging around the hotel, I threw away the frozen bag of peas and bought a one-way train ticket from Rutland to Baltimore. The shoulder wasn't feeling better. Lying in bed at night with my arm in a fixed position resulted in sporadic bouts of restless sleep. I was fatigued and still angry with myself for being so careless. It was time to go home. Ignominiously, I had been felled by a tree bump, not even a tree stump.

On the ride home from the train station, I gave Brite the details about the fall and the hospital visit.

"I figured it was more serious than what you were telling me," she said with a sheepish grin.

"But it shouldn't have ended like this. I was three quarters of the way to Katahdin. I feel like I failed," I said dejectedly, my voice trailing off.

"Just remember what you told me back in Georgia when I left the trail," she reminded me gently.

"Yeah, yeah, I know. I didn't quit. The mountain just told me to go home," I replied half-heartedly.

"Who knows, maybe we can get you back on the trail quicker than you think." I loved Brite's enthusiastic optimism, but we both knew the odds were not in my favor.

Transitioning from the trail was more difficult than I had expected. I was depressed, demoralized, and utterly defeated. For the first week, I woke up in the middle of the night in a panicked daze as if I were lost in the darkness. Nothing was familiar. I was a stranger in my own house. Was this how my father felt at the nursing home? Behind the wheel of a car, I felt like a teenager with a learner's permit. Measuring miles in minutes instead of hours was a strange sensation.

Meanwhile, the transition to home-cooked meals was effortless. I needed to eat as much as possible. Since Springer Mountain, I had lost nearly forty pounds, almost 20% of my body weight. I weighed 156 pounds. I hadn't weighed that little since high school. My upper body had also lost considerable muscle mass. Brite correctly noted that I had the chest of a ten-year-old boy. Since Connecticut, I had been using foam rubber pads to tighten my backpack around my chest.

The MRI revealed an AC ligament tear and smaller tears in my rotator cuff. The numerous falls on the shoulder and the constant pulling motion involved with climbing had taken its toll. Even though my shoulder was feeling better, there was no way I could continue the hike without risking complete tears to the frayed tissue. Treatment was rest and physical therapy. Even with the knee healing quickly, Herm's Hike was hiking history. There was no way to reach Baxter State Park before it closed on October 15.

I updated my trail journal with the headline: "Sunset on Sondance (for this season)!" Only two weeks earlier, I announced with "Thud in Vermud!" that I might be sidelined temporarily. In my final journal entry for the year, I thanked my supporters for opening up their hearts, homes, and wallets.

Over the ensuing days, my mood lightened as e-mails of support flooded my mailbox. Lisa and members from the Dalton United Methodist Church reminded me that my fall in the mountains was not a fall from grace. Every action in our lives had a purpose, even if we failed to see the connection. I was home because I needed to be with my father and family. In my new state of perpetual being, my presence in the lives of others was God's presence. I was sure that B would agree with my new definition of being.

Bluebird reminded me to be proud of my accomplishment. Reluctantly, I had to agree. I had raised just over $5,000 for the Alzheimer's Association, almost $3 per mile. Although far short of my goal of 10K, it was an impressive total for a grassroots fundraiser.

Just as amazing, I hiked nearly 1,700 miles with two surgically repaired feet, two surgically repaired shoulders, and two surgically repaired wrists. Instead of being held together with baling wire and bubblegum, I was held together with plastic staples and titanium screws. Not too bad for someone over the hill but still not over the last mountain.

Chapter 22
An Old Soldier Fades Away
(Parkton, MD)

My first weekend home, I ditched the arm sling (not wanting to worry any family members) and visited my father with Brite. As we entered the room, he briefly glanced at us as if passing strangers on the street. His face was gaunt; his body emaciated; his skin desiccated. The disease was rapidly advancing and severing more connections in the brain with ruthless abandonment. At meals, he pecked weakly and blindly at his food like a baby bird.

His eyes were cloudy and colorless like old glass. I wondered what he saw. Was he able to peer beyond this earthly plane and peek into heaven? I remembered the times during his first year in the nursing home when he called out to deceased family members around his bed. Who's to say he didn't see them?

Despite the overwhelming sadness that shrouded the room, there was always a ray of sunshine with my mother's arrival. Upon seeing my mother enter the room, my father would perk up for a brief second or two. His eyes would sparkle and a bemused grin would gently stretch across his face. In a raspy, unintelligible whisper, he would attempt to call out her name while trying to raise his arms for a hug. Alzheimer's could eradicate the brain, but it could never extinguish the gift of transcendent love, even as the symptoms worsened.

I quickly settled into my pre-hike routine. Twice a week and on Sundays, I chauffeured my mother back and forth to the nursing home. If Brite wasn't with me, I usually returned to spend time alone with my father. Since my father could no longer speak, we spent most of our time watching television while I held his hand. I don't know how much my father saw or heard, but he was attracted to the bright colors and moving images like an infant.

On one occasion, I brought along my portable CD/cassette player in a last-ditch effort to spark a memory. I popped in a CD, but my father sat motionless. The music had lost its magic.

In 2007 music had been a magic elixir. I didn't need medical experts to tell me that Alzheimer's patients connected with music, especially with music buried in their long-term memory. Music from the '40s and '50s was the soundtrack of my father's life, and Frank Sinatra was the crooner.

Seconds after pushing the "play" button, my father and his roommate Paul, who was blind and bedridden, would start singing robustly whatever lyrics they could muster. They were off key and out of tune like two drunken sailors, but it didn't matter. For a few minutes, I heard the happiness in their voices as they relived some sweet memory from a distant past when they were young and life was full of promise.

Often when my mother and I were visiting, my

father would suddenly burst into song. Usually, the tune was "The Way You Look Tonight" or "My Way." Other popular songs on my father's song list were "Here I Am Lord" and "How Are Things in Glocca Morra," the song about a fictional village in Ireland from the 1947 musical *Finian's Rainbow*. The Catholic hymn I could understand, but "Glocca Morra" was a mystery. Maybe Geralyn from Kent was right. Somewhere in my father's genetic makeup, there were a few rogue Irish genes dancing about.

The sight of my father singing always brought a smile to my mother's face. Like other family members, she was mystified at my father's sudden singing career until I confessed to being the session producer.

Since my father ate and drank very little, it was just a matter of time until he succumbed to the disease. Often I witnessed my mother holding his hand and tenderly whispering in his ear, "Herman, listen to me, my sweetheart. You can let go now. It's your time. There's no reason for you to stay. We're (the family) going to be fine." I always left the room with tears in my eyes. His will to love was the will to live, but it was only a matter of time before the spirit surrendered the body.

At 9:46 p.m. on November 17, my sister called and said that Dad had passed away. Brite and I were the first family members to arrive at the nursing home. My father was lying in bed with his hands folded over his chest. I sat down next to my father and gripped his still warm hands. "Thank you, Dad, for being a good father. I hope that I was a good son," I whispered hoarsely as tears streamed down my cheeks. I leaned over the bed and gently kissed him on his forehead.

For a few minutes, I stood in silence and gazed upon my father's countenance. I watched in amazement as the creases and folds in his face miraculously receded. The disease was wearily releasing its stranglehold. For a brief second, I saw a peaceful smile that said, "It's okay. I'm fine. Don't worry about me." I smiled back through the tears. Exhausted, my father had finally fallen on the battlefield of life. He died victorious as a soldier of Christ as he would have wanted.

On Monday morning at the funeral home, my sister placed a small wooden sailboat inside the casket during the final viewing. My father often talked about buying a sailboat and sailing to the islands in the Pacific Ocean. Perhaps, that dream was the chance to retrieve his youthful innocence that had been obliterated by the Japanese attack on Pearl Harbor.

"Fair winds and following seas, you noble mariner, you mystic voyager," I whispered. Someday we would meet across the boundless expanse of the universe that separated us like a great ocean. Together in spirit, we would walk over the distant horizon toward that new dawn that I had promised my nephew. Inside the limousine, I wondered if my father remembered those prophetic words he boldly proclaimed about the AT over fifty years ago.

Inside the church vestibule, the American flag was removed from the casket and replaced with a pall, the white garment that symbolized my father's baptism. My oldest daughter, dressed in her Coast Guard uniform with white gloves, escorted the casket to the front of the altar. Once the pallbearers were seated, she walked to the head of the casket and stood at attention. With her head angled slightly down, she deliberately stepped around the casket for a final inspection. At one point, she stopped to ceremoniously straighten a corner of the pall. Returning to the front of the casket, she rendered a farewell salute, slowly raising her right hand before slowly returning it to the side. Wiping a tear from my eye, I imagined my father looking down from heaven, beaming with pride.

After Communion, my youngest daughter, a biology and classical voice major, sang "Ave Maria." Accompanied by a pianist, her soprano soared beyond the rafters. No heavenly choir of angels could have sounded better. My financial investment in voice, piano, and cello lessons had paid off handsomely. If my daughter never sang another song again, my money had been well spent.

Before Mass concluded, I delivered the eulogy. Since Springer Mountain, I had been preparing for this moment, often composing snippets in the stillness of nature as I walked the trail alone. With heavy feet and a heavier heart, I nervously climbed the steps to the pulpit. No climb on the trail had been more difficult. I gazed down at family and friends as if standing on a mountaintop. I was ready to deliver the speech of a lifetime, my father's lifetime.

I recalled my father's childhood during the Great Depression, his WWII experience, and his heroic battle with Alzheimer's disease. A humble and compassionate man, my father endured his illness with a spiritual grace that reflected an inner peace and inspired all of those around him. However, during those dark nights of the soul, the ghosts of a faraway battlefield would silently drift across his mind. The nursing staff often heard him barking out orders and shouting out the names of forgotten soldiers. The brutal combat and the death of his men were burdens that my father carried to the grave.

I concluded the eulogy with these words: "In dying, he taught us how to live. In living, he taught us how to love. To live and to love is a life well spoken. What a wonderful legacy for an old soldier who never died but just faded away." I had no more words to say about my hero.

At the gravesite service in the cold rain, the honor guard fired a rifle volley and "Taps" was sounded. The flag on the casket was folded and presented to my mother by my daughter. With the service ended, a bagpiper on a distant knoll played "Amazing Grace." Accompanied by Brite and my daughters arm in arm, I walked away feeling as if a great weight had been lifted from my shoulders. The last page in my father's book of life had been written. It was now time to celebrate that story with family and friends.

Over Thanksgiving and Christmas, I was constantly asked when I would be returning to the trail. I was ambivalent. Physically, I was fine, but mentally, I was still exhausted. The inner fire had been doused. People didn't realize the staggering physical and mental effort it took to hike the AT. The mountains heal but they also hurt.

Brite and my mother strongly encouraged me to return. "Don't be a popsicle," they exhorted in my father's words. In the end, they finally convinced me that Herm's Hike was now Herm and Paul's hike. That's what my father would have wanted. That was my healing moment. Like Aliyah in Franklin, it was time to move forward until I ran out of white blazes.

After announcing my decision to return, I shared a secret story with Brite and my mother. The night my father died, I returned home around midnight and walked outside to decompress and collect my thoughts. It was a cold, crisp, and clear November night. The sky was filled with millions of twinkling stars. Every few steps, I stopped and stared despairingly at the heavens. Before heading inside, I stopped one last time. "Just a sign, Pop, someday, somewhere, and somehow," I whispered forlornly. Seconds later, a shooting star, maybe two stars, exploded in space and rocketed to the east and the north. "North. That's the direction I need to be heading," I said softly with a tight grin. More dots had been connected. The cosmic portrait was coming into focus, but there were more dots waiting on the trail.

Chapter 23
Eagle Man and the Sacred Stone
(Parkton to Billings, MT)

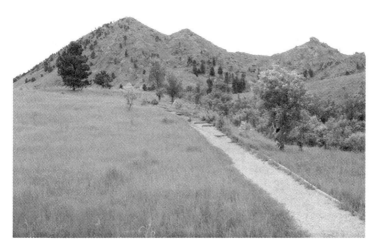

Trailhead to the sacred Bear Butte. Notice prayer flags and bundles on tree to the right.

Before returning to the trail, Brite and I traveled to Montana for a family wedding. Being retired with no time constraints, we decided on a road trip of a lifetime. Beyond the Mississippi River, we seemed to be following a path of invisible white blazes. Stopping in Iowa to visit Brite's brother, we spent an afternoon at the Field of Dreams (site of the baseball field in the eponymous movie) in Dyersville where we played in a pick-up game and talked baseball with the fans. Instead of flashbacks to the movie, I was reliving my day at Backer Park.

Crossing into South Dakota, we hiked up Spirit Mound, one of the few verifiable sites where explorers Meriwether Lewis and William Clark stopped on the greatest road trip in American history. From the seventy-foot bedrock knob, we watched an ocean of prairie grasses sway in the wind like an endless wave. Local Sioux tribes believed evil spirits known as the "Little People" inhabited the mountain. That legend reminded me of the "Little People" of the Cherokees. The mound proved that all mountains, no matter how high, were filled with myth and magic, and all tribes in the family of mankind were connected.

Three days later, we stopped at the Crazy Horse Memorial on our way to Mount Rushmore. In 1948, sculptor Korczak Ziolkowski was commissioned by Lakota elder Henry Standing Bear to depict the Oglala Lakota warrior on horseback as the Native Americans response to Mount Rushmore. After a lifetime of sculpting the mountain, Korczak, who in his later years looked like the Polish version of Grizzly Adams, died in 1992. With his death, the family inherited the ongoing project. Throughout its history, the nonprofit entity adamantly and proudly accepted no government money. The Great White Father would have no claim or connection to the mountain or the men, Crazy Horse and Korczak.

After a bus ride to the foot of the mountain, Brite

and I returned to browse through the memorial complex. In the hallways, American Native artists and artisans were busy selling their goods. Being a bibliophile, I was immediately attracted to a book table where I picked up the closest book to peruse. On the back cover was a photo of the author. I looked at the picture and then glanced at the gentleman behind the table.

"You're the author. Semper Fi," I exclaimed, always eager to meet a writer.

"Semper Fi. I'm Ed McGaa, Eagle Man," he replied with a firm handshake. After introducing ourselves, we engaged in small talk about his books. Other than being marines and authors, it didn't appear that we had anything else in common. That quickly changed once I started talking about Herm's Hike.

"What's your trail name?" Ed asked, obviously familiar with hiking customs.

"Sondance," I replied. Ed looked bemused and irritated.

"Sun Dance as in the Oglala sacred ceremony?" he asked in a serious tone.

"No, Sondance as in the good son who dances with the mountain to honor the father," I replied, hoping my comments were not offensive. For the first time, I realized the other association with my trail name. How could I have forgotten? The movie *A Man Called Horse*, which I had seen in college, had dramatically depicted a "Hollywood version" of the ceremony. After reciting the story about the origin of my trail name and Herm's Hike, Ed broke into a smile and nodded his head in agreement.

"And where has your journey taken you since you left home?" he asked.

"Spirit Mound, Saint Joseph's Indian School, The Badlands, Pine Ridge Reservation, Wounded Knee, and today the Crazy Horse Monument and Rushmore. Hopefully, Little Bighorn and Devil's Tower before Billings," I replied.

"Why the interest in Indian culture if you're not a pretendian, a wasichu?" Ed asked somewhat sarcastically, having met his fair share of Indian wannabes.

After speaking about the need for Americans to rediscover, or in most cases discover, their history, I got down to the heart of the matter. "There's one undeniable truth I learned while hiking the Appalachian Trail. To enhance your relationship with God, you do it through the divinity of nature. Native Americans had a direct relationship with God through the natural world, and that's what people should be seeking today. That legacy of your people could be a path of spirituality for modern man," I stated dramatically.

Ed leaned slightly forward and stared hard into my eyes as if peering into my soul. He couldn't believe what his ears had just heard. "You, my friend, are not on a vacation. You are on a spiritual journey. The Great Spirit has brought us together for a reason," he pronounced with a twinkle in his eye.

Before leaving, Ed placed his hand on my shoulder and prayed over me in his native tongue for my safe journey on the hike. I didn't understand a word, but I didn't need to. The reverence and emotion in his voice gave me goose bumps. I was honored to be the recipient of such a prayer.

"Sondance, you must go to the sacred mountain at Bear Butte. Do this as a personal favor for me," he said solemnly. I readily agreed, knowing that my promise was now a sacred oath with the Great Spirit. Besides that, when Ed spoke, you listened.

Born on the Pine Ridge Reservation, Ed was a registered tribal member of the Oglala Sioux. At age seventeen, he enlisted in the US Marine Corps during the Korean War. After graduating from college, he returned to Officer Candidate School and became a marine fighter pilot. Following 110 missions during the Vietnam War, he returned home to a hero's welcome from his people. He had participated in the Sun Dance ceremony six times and authored twelve books on Indian culture, religion, and spirituality.

Later that afternoon, Brite and I visited Mount Rushmore. Compared to the Crazy Horse Monument, this tribute to the four Great White Fathers was austere and sterile. Built on sacred land of the Lakota in the Black Hills, I found the ostentatious tourist trap an insult to Native Americans. My talk with Ed, who had commented that Rushmore would be like having a statue of Hitler outside Auschwitz, had affected me. Like Ed, I now saw Mount Rushmore as a monument to the US government's systemized genocide of the Native Americans, a reminder of the darkest chapter in American history. Perhaps, for that reason alone, I surmised that it should stand for eternity.

The next day Brite and I headed to Bear Butte. Visible from miles away, the geological formation, resembling a sleeping bear, had a magnetic pull on my spirit. Rising 4,426 feet above sea level like a church steeple, the mountain was a holy site for the Plains Indians. Today it remained a pilgrimage for Native Americans where religious ceremonies were frequently conducted.

Before heading to the trailhead, we stopped at the visitor/education center to pick up some literature about hiking the sacred mountain. Other than a handful of park staff, we were the only visitors at the time. Outside the building, we admired the bust of Frank Fools Crow, Eagle Man's spiritual mentor and spiritual advisor.

As we climbed the steep trail, we marveled at the hundreds of brightly colored prayer clothes and tobacco ties fluttering in the hot wind. The vivid colors contrasted sharply to the bleak terrain. In 1996, a fire destroyed most of the trees on the mountain. In its wake, it left a charred and scarred landscape of black and gray sentinels that reminded me of the gray ghosts on Clingmans Dome. At the summit, Brite and I enjoyed an eagle's-eye view of the endless prairie as if we were riding the thermals.

Back in the parking lot, an older gentleman approached Brite and me. Dressed in a dark green work shirt, he appeared to be a park employee. "Mike Red Feather," he said, extending his hand. "You folks are a long way from home. Mind if I ask what brings you to our mountain?" Obviously, he had seen our license plate.

"We're headed to Billings for a wedding, but yesterday we met Eagle Man at the Crazy Horse Monument. He told us we should stop here and hike the sacred mountain," I replied in a friendly manner, not sure if Red Feather was one of the native panhandlers that Eagle Man said to avoid.

"Great warrior, the Eagle Man. I can see that you're hikers," he said, pointing to the AT sticker on the rear window. "If there's anything I can do for you while you're here, just let me know."

"Well, now that you mentioned it. There is one thing," I said haltingly, not sure how my request would be received. "I need a flat rock about six-by-twelve inches to place on Mount Katahdin when I finish my hike. I need something symbolic of my journey that has some spiritual meaning," I added before explaining Herm's Hike.

"A wotai stone like the Eagle Man carried in battle to protect him from harm," he mused.

"No, nothing that sacred or personal. Just a rock from the mountain," I added, not wanting to appear like a pretendian. Eagle Man had told me the story about his wotai stone, a type of guardian angel, and how it had saved him from being shot down numerous times. I could readily relate. In some ways, I carried my own wotai stones in my backpack for protection: my father's dog tag, his unit patch, my aunt's prayers card, and Brite's love notes.

"All the rocks from the mountain are sacred, lelah wah ste wakan (very holy and very spiritual)," he remarked. "Wait here for a minute. I'll be right back."

Red Feather disappeared behind the center and reappeared with a flat rock cradled in his hands.

"A gift from my people to you, but with one condition. If you do not place this rock at the top of Mount Katahdin, you must return it here," he said piously before handing me the sacred stone.

"Pilaymaya (Thank you). I will see that it gets to its rightful place," I said humbly, gently reaching for the rock with a slight bow.

"Wakan Takan kici un. May the Great Spirit bless you," he said solemnly as we both held the rock before he lifted it toward my chest.

As our visitor walked away, Brite and I carefully examined the gift. Medium gray in color with flecks of glittering white and silver, it was the perfect rock for Mount Katahdin. Now all I had to do was get it there. If not, I wondered how much it would cost to mail a rock back to the park. With my luck, I would have the postal inspectors and the FBI hot on my trail for smuggling Indian artifacts across interstate lines.

On the road to Billings, I pondered the impromptu meeting with Red Feather. Had Eagle Man contacted Red Feather to be on the lookout for two hiking palefaces? I was tempted to turn around and head back to the park office, but decided against it. In the words of Eagle Man, mysteries of the Great Spirit are best left unknown. Embrace the mystery and accept them as proof of his presence.

My imagination ran wild as I envisioned Red Feather as a visitor from the spirit world. I could see the staff at Bear Butte saying, "Never heard of anybody named Red Feather, and by the way, give us the rock back."

The next day Brite and I stopped at Sundance, Wyoming, for lunch. Named after the sacred dance, the town also laid claim to the outlaw Harry Longabaugh. While serving time in the Cook County jail for stealing a horse, Longabaugh adopted the nickname the Sundance Kid. Outside the former jail, there was a statue of the outlaw lounging on a bench inside his cell. While Brite clicked away, I posed for a few shots with my namesake.

Four days after the wedding, Brite and I returned home to prepare for the hike. As I readied my gear, I couldn't help thinking that I had never left the trail. For me, the white blazes had extended west to an author's table at the Crazy Horse Monument. I wondered if the trail would ever end.

Chapter 24

Ver-mud and Ver-done in Vermont

(Rutland, VT, to Lincoln, NH)

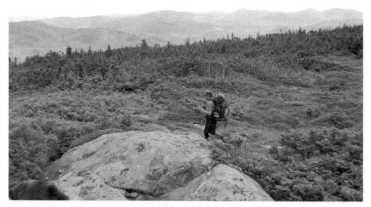

Trekking across a mountain plateau, New England's answer to the balds. Hiking at its finest.

On Monday, June 28, I rode the rails back to Rutland with nervous anticipation. Physically I was fully healed. Had I healed mentally and emotionally? That was the question to be answered. Tomorrow morning on the trail,

I would have that answer. Heading north out of New York, the AMTRAK coach was packed with businessmen dressed in wingtip shoes, button-down shirts, and club ties, looking as I did in high school. Standing out from the crowd in shorts and a t-shirt with a backpack, I became a topic of conversation. As we approached Albany, Jack, who was sitting next to me, stood up and announced a collection was being taken for the Alzheimer's Association and Herm's Hike. When my ball cap was returned, it contained $72. It felt good to be on the road again. Any doubts about returning to the trail had evaporated.

I arrived in Rutland at around 9 p.m. and walked across the street to the Back Home Again Café. "Back home again on the trail," I muttered to myself cheerfully. The restaurant was closed, but the hostel was open. I was welcome to any leftovers in the kitchen.

At breakfast, I heard a shofar reverberate throughout the building and was invited to morning prayer with the staff. We hurriedly gathered upstairs and formed a prayer circle. After a scripture reading, we went around the room to give thanks. When it came to my turn, I paraphrased the parable of the Good Samaritan. "I want to thank you for allowing me to bear witness to Jesus Christ through your charity," I said sincerely, remembering the Amish family on Clingmans Dome. From the nodding of heads, my comments had been well received. Before leaving, I was invited to the farm but politely declined. I had a trail to hike.

Later that morning, the shuttle dropped me off at the parking lot to Thundering Falls. I walked back to the trail where Don found me last year. Although curious about the stump, there was no need to return to the accident scene. I was focused on the present, not the past. I took my first step north under a bright sunny sky with temperatures in the low 70s. Once again, I was one with the mountain, one with nature. The trees cheered my return.

For two days, I had the trail to myself, one of the benefits of being an early NOBO. I averaged about fifteen miles a day for the three-day hike through the Vermont lowlands where the highest peak was just over 2,600 feet. Late afternoon on day three, I crossed the Connecticut River and walked up the hill to Hanover, New Hampshire, home of Dartmouth College. Vermont, or Ver-mud, call it what you want, it was Ver-done. Now there were only two states left. It was still way too early to start counting the remaining miles, but last year's fall was a distant memory.

The sidewalks were overflowing with preppie parents and students. Needing a break, I bought an ice cream cone and sat on a bench next to a middle-aged couple who were dressed for the golf course. As I licked away enjoying the human parade, I noticed the woman glancing at the backpack.

"Are you a student here, if you don't mind me asking?" she asked haughtily.

"No, just a hiker passing through here, if you don't mind me answering," I chirped before explaining how the AT ran through downtown Hanover. The couple had just dropped off their daughter for freshman orientation.

"Where do you eat and sleep?" the woman inquired in the same cavalier tone.

"It's all here in my backpack, freeze-dried meals, tent, sleeping bag," I replied.

"Aren't you a little old for this kind of thing?" she

asked incredulously.

"Yes, I am, but I'm not out here alone," I remarked proudly before making my sales pitch about Herm's Hike. After I had finished, the woman fished a ten-dollar bill out of her purse and handed it to me.

"Good luck to you, Paul, or Sondance, or whatever you call yourself out there. I admire your tenacity," she wisecracked before leaving. It was no surprise that Dartmouth's school colors were green and white. Like the mountain ski slopes, the streets were filled with a lot of white people with a lot of greenbacks.

I hiked through the town and spent the night at Tigger's Tree House, a private residence with two RVs and a club basement for use by hikers. After dinner, I watched *Field of Dreams* in the privacy of my own class B camper. The hike was off to a great start.

The next morning my streak of good weather ended in a cloudburst. Once the rain stopped, the temperature soared to the low 90s. With the heat and humidity, every insect in the universe suddenly rose from the earth in a steamy cloud of biblical proportions. The forest had become a sweltering tropical jungle. Within an hour, my sweat-wicking shirt and shorts were soaked in a heavy sweat that fermented with each passing minute. By midday, I smelled like vomit. At one point, I hiked naked for about a mile, thinking that it would stop the sweating. To my disbelief and discomfort, I seemed to sweat even more without clothes. Unknowingly, I had gone from one of the wettest summers in New England last year to one of the hottest.

Having seen only a handful of hikers the entire day, I was delighted to find two other hikers at the shelter that evening. One was Tadpole, a young man in his late twenties from Austin, Texas, who had worked for eight years as a roadie for Willie Nelson. Both of his parents, who were lifelong employees of Willie, had finally convinced him to find a more suitable career. Earlier in the year, he quit the band and hit the trail. After his hike, he planned to return to college and study landscape architecture. Throughout the evening, he regaled us with tales from the road, declaring that most of the tabloid stories about Willie were true. When Tadpole's mother died from brain cancer a few years ago, Willie paid all of her hospital bills.

Story time ended with a thunderstorm that stretched until dawn. Sleep was fitful. A couple of times I had to move my sleeping bag away from the leaky roof. The following morning, a pair of hiking boots left outside was filled to the brim with rainwater. All we could do was laugh. Gore-Tex worked both ways.

The following morning I stopped at the home of Bill Ackerly, a retired psychiatrist known as the Ice Cream Man. As I stepped up to the house decorated with icicle lights and Tibetan prayer flags, Bill was busy greeting hikers and handing out ice cream sandwiches. Instead of a morning coffee, I had a morning ice cream. I left Bill's place with a new tribe of section hikers: three from Germany with backpacks that resembled small refrigerators, and a couple from Texas, named Hobo and Variable. Of course, Hobo wasn't a real hobo much to my disappointment, but Variable was a math teacher.

From Bill's place to the summit of Smarts Mountain, the elevation gain was over 2,500 feet in four miles. It was my biggest mountain since Killington last year. Progress was slow but steady in the heat.

With one false peak after another, the mountain was mentally exhausting. As I climbed up the last section of rebar steps, thunder boomed in the distance. Looking over my shoulder, I saw a massive dark cloud rushing toward us like a tidal wave. I immediately quickened my pace, leaving the others behind. I wanted to get to the fire warden's cabin on the summit as soon as possible.

On the summit plateau, a cold rain started to fall. Just as I reached the front porch of the cabin, a gale blew over the peak with a deafening roar. Within minutes, the temperature fell nearly forty degrees. Marble-sized hail strafed the dilapidated cabin like machine-gun fire. Hikers crowded the doorway to watch nature's fury, hoping the cabin would withstand the barrage. I only hoped that my tribe members weren't too far behind me.

While the storm raged outside, I battled it inside. While eating a snack, I began to shiver. I quickly changed into a dry shirt and put on my rain jacket for warmth. By the time I zipped up the jacket, my teeth were chattering and my body was shaking uncontrollably. I yanked out my down-filled sleeping bag and crawled quickly inside. Still shivering violently, someone threw an open sleeping bag on top of me. Fifteen minutes later, I was sitting up and resting comfortably with a cup of hot chocolate, courtesy of a fellow hiker. As a rosy hue returned to my skin, the rest of my tribe trudged wearily into the cabin. When the hail started, they sought shelter underneath a tree and huddled together under their tent footprints.

Opting for more floor space, I hiked to the next shelter later in the afternoon. That evening at dinner, everyone swapped stories about the storm. "Man, we were really worried about you. Your face was pale white and your breathing was shallow," said one of the hikers who attended to me at the cabin. Their compassion was the bond of brotherhood held sacred by all hikers. Silently, I promised to "pay it forward," but I was worried. I hadn't fared well with my first big mountain, and the biggest ones were ahead.

The following morning I was on the trail at daylight, eager to put yesterday behind me. For five miles, I walked alone in silent contemplation. Yesterday my sleeping bag, the Phantom 800, may have saved my life instead of my backpack. Had my spirit guide switched from an osprey to a phantom, from an animal to an apparition? It was another silly thought that helped pass the miles, part of the mind game on the AT.

Reaching the first road crossing of the day at NH 25, I stopped to sit on a boulder in the parking lot and imagine an egg sandwich and a fresh cup of coffee in the village of Wentworth. What I couldn't imagine was walking five miles to town along a deserted country road. With plenty of food and water, the only thing to do was to keep hiking.

Waiting to cross the road, a black pickup truck screeched to a stop and backed up to where I was standing. "Man, you look like you could use a friend or a cup of coffee. Get in. I know where you can find both," the driver bellowed. I quickly threw the backpack into the bed of the truck, noting the Marine Corps sticker on the bumper, and climbed into the passenger's side.

"Semper Fi. Paul Travers or Sondance as I'm known on the trail," I said gleefully, extending my right hand.

"Semper Fi, buddy! I'm John Thompson, but you

can call me Big John," the man crowed with a hearty belly laugh. With his crew cut, weathered face that looked like an old bulldog, and calloused hands the size of oven mitts, Big John lived up to his name. A combat marine in the Korean Conflict, he returned home after the war to start a tree service and logging operation. He was an avid outdoorsman who loved to hike and hunt the mountains.

"I guess I was born about a hundred years too late for my liking," Big John exclaimed wistfully as we pulled into the parking lot of Shawnee's General Store.

Inside Big John made a beeline for the coffee counter before heading for a bench in front of the store with a tray of coffee cups. John introduced me to his friends, a group of retirees who had gathered for their weekly bull session.

"Hey, Big John, what about me? I'm retired. Where's my coffee?" I joked as everyone started sipping.

"Now you just march back in there and get what you want. Tell them to put it on Big John's tab," he replied.

"Tell them to put it on Cheap John's tab," one the gang shouted amid a roar of laughter.

I rejoined the group with a breakfast sandwich and a fresh cup of coffee, taking a seat next to Big John. For the next hour, I learned everything about everybody who had ever lived in Wentworth.

At one point, an older woman in a sundress pedaled by the store on a vintage bicycle with a bell and basket filled with flowers. Big John nudged me in the ribs. "What do you think about that beauty, Paul? That's one fine, good-looking woman," John said, smacking his lips in a romantic fantasy.

"A classic beauty, Big John. I bet she was quite a

looker in her younger days," I replied cautiously, caught off guard by the comment.

"You have fine taste in women, Paul, because that's my wife. I think she rides by here to check up on me," Big John roared above the laughter from his cronies.

An hour and a half later, Big John dropped me off at the trailhead. Later that afternoon, I arrived at the Hikers Welcome Hostel. Just a short walk from the trail, the two-story wood structure was spacious and comfortably cluttered with hiking gear, books, magazines, old furniture, and a wall of DVDs, one of the best collections on the trail.

That evening, I dined with two other hikers at the Green Wood Restaurant. My young and brash dinner partners had come for the Moosilauke Challenge. To win the contest and a free meal, two people had to consume an eight-pound pizza, named the Moosilauke Monster, in less than ninety minutes. Ninety-one minutes later, the contestants stood up from the table and returned to the hostel with almost three pounds of pizza.

That evening the leftover pizza made a great snack for watching movies. The featured film was *The Big Lebowski*, a comedy starring Jeff Bridges as the Dude, a burned-out hippie slacker; and John Goodman as Walter, a psychotic burned-out Vietnam vet whose life was bowling. Filled with drug references and sex scenes reminiscent of the late '60s, I laughed until tears ran down my face. The younger hikers liked it so much that we watched it twice, but they didn't find it as funny as I did. "I grew up with guys like this," I howled when questioned about my unbridled hilarity.

The more we watched, the more beer we drank,

and the more Phatt Chapp, one of the caretakers, started to look like a young John Goodman. Whenever Goodman appeared on the screen, we'd glance at Phatt Chapp, shout "Walter," and laugh even harder.

I didn't know if Phatt Chapp realized he was the brunt of a good-natured joke, but the next day when someone called him Walter, he laughed along with us.

The next morning, the pizza contestants and I pooled our money to slackpack Mount Moosilauke from the north. At 4,802 feet, the mountain was the portal to the Whites and offered a glimpse of the trail all the way to Mount Katahdin. After a short walk from the trailhead, we climbed 2,000 feet in a mile and a half next to the Beaver Brook Cascades. Being next to a waterfall, the trail was a slippery ladder of rock ledges, wood steps, and metal rungs. One misstep could result in a tumble down the mountain or the waterfall.

As we climbed higher, the light drizzle became a steady rain. Above the tree line, a howling wind was blowing the freezing rain sideways in a heavy fog. I pulled the drawstrings on my jacket hood as tight as I could, leaned forward, and turned my face away from the wind. After a brief rest stop at the summit, once the site of a resort hotel, we hustled to the opposite tree line. At the bottom of the mountain, we were greeted by a sunny summer day. Today Mother Nature warned us to be prepared for the mountains. I was listening intently. Welcome to the Whites!

Starting from Kinsman Notch the next day by myself, I hiked the winding ridge from South Kinsman Mountain to North Kinsman Mountain, both peaks near 4,300 feet, in the cold rain. My prelude to the great sights in the Whites was hidden behind a curtain of clouds. I hoped it wasn't a harbinger of mountains to come.

Reaching Lonesome Lake Hut, I stopped for a cup of coffee and a chance to get out of the rain. This was the first of eight cabins operated by the Appalachian Mountain Club (AMC) for vacation hikers. Staffed by college kids known as the croo, the paying customer received dinner, nightly entertainment, a bunk, and breakfast. Being one of the early NOBOs, I looked forward to work-for-stay opportunities. For an hour or two of menial labor, such as sweeping floors or washing dishes, thru-hikers received a sleeping space indoors and a hearty meal of any leftovers.

At Franconia Notch where the trail crossed US 3 and I-93, I reached a major crossroad that defined my hike. Do I hike another two plus miles to a tent site or hitch a ride into town? Remembering the advice of Brite and my mother, it was time for Paul's Hike. I had promised myself to listen to the trail and let it lead me. Today that little voice in my head whispered, "Go to Lincoln."

"Not much room in here, but if you don't mind holding your backpack in your lap, I'll give you a ride," Jason announced cheerfully. Every inch of his Subaru station wagon was crammed with camping gear, photo equipment, and duck decoys.

A recent college graduate, Jason decided to pursue his childhood dream and photograph the loon for a book. He sank all of his money into camping gear and hi-tech cameras and hit the road. The lakes and ponds of New England would be his home for the rest of the summer and the fall. He had no set itinerary and no timetable. Tonight his home was going to be a mountain lake somewhere in the White Mountain National Forest.

Jason dropped me off in front of a Dunkin' Donuts. "Thanks for the nature lesson and keep following your dream," I said sincerely. After giving me directions to Chet's Place, he headed north. Looking around, I couldn't help but notice the signs for Loon Mountain Ski Resort. Jason and I had a lot in common when it came to pursuing childhood dreams on the road.

After a cup of coffee and a couple of chocolate doughnuts, I walked to Chet's Place. In the driveway of the quaint rancher, three people were talking, one of them in a wheelchair. "Chet's place?' I asked, having spotted the carved bear and the AT sign on the front lawn.

"You found it and I'm Chet," said the young man in the wheelchair. "Go inside and make yourself comfortable. I'll be with you in a few minutes."

Minutes later, Chet and his assistant Fallon gave me the grand tour of the hostel that was a garage version of Hikers Welcome Hostel. After a hot shower, I plopped down on the couch and reached for the binder on the coffee table titled *Chet's Story*. Curious about my host, I opened the binder, immediately spellbound. The collection of newspaper articles chronicled Chet's incredible journey from avid outdoorsman to hostel owner.

In 2001, while preparing for his own AT hike, Chet was set on fire when his new camp stove exploded. He was medevaced to Massachusetts General Hospital where he spent over eight months in a drug-induced coma. He suffered multiple major organ failures and flatlined nine times. His lungs were permanently scarred from the toxic smoke and flames. His midsection received third-degree burns that destroyed a significant amount of muscle tissue. Miraculously, his face and arms were unscathed by the fire. After eighteen months in the hospital, the Miracle Man (as he was dubbed by the New England media) was discharged. In 2007, wanting to stay active in the hiking community, he used settlement money from the stove's manufacturer to open a hostel that was appropriately named One Step at a Time. "One step at a time" had been the mantra from my guardian angel on Clingmans Dome.

Later that evening I sat down and talked with Chet about my hike, his hostel, and his battle to return to a normal life. When I mentioned my father's conversation with dead relatives in the nursing home, Chet related his own harrowing tale in the afterlife after flatlining.

"I was standing in front of a doorway where a blinding light was shining from the other side. Gradually, I started to see the faces of loved ones. When I tried to step across to the other side, they told me to go back because it wasn't my time," he said softly with tears in his eyes. At that moment, he recognized there was a purpose for his life. His challenge was to discover and embrace it. Chet downplayed any comments about his inspirational courage, proclaiming that he was more inspired by those he met from the trail. I then told him about Jenna in Hot Springs.

"I'll have to get down there one day. I'd love to meet her. Inspiration like a cloud comes in all shapes and sizes," he mused with a soft smile. *Love like a cloud comes in all shapes and size*, I pondered quietly, thinking back to my meeting with Jenna's mom in Hot Springs.

Chapter 25
Knights in the Whites
(Lincoln to Carlo Col Shelter, ME)

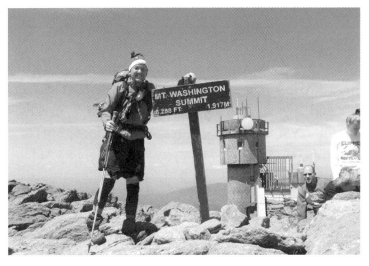

A rare, sunny day on Mount Washington but still windy and cold.

That next morning I rode back to Franconia Notch with one of Chet's friends. Within minutes, I was quickly reminded that the Appalachian Trail was really the Appalachian Mountain Trail. The climb to the first peak at Little Haystack Mountain (elevation at 4,800 feet) was nearly 2,500 feet over two and a half miles with rock climbs, rock steps, and rock scrambles.

As I moved higher, the forest changed from hardwoods to evergreens. At the sight of stunted firs and spruces, I quickened my pace with excitement. The summit was near. Emerging from the tree line, I stopped dead in my tracks, breathless and speechless. Before me stretched a mountain ridgeline trail that extended for nearly fifty miles.

I was spellbound. These were the mountains of my dreams since Georgia. These were my Himalayas. I was king of the mountain, just an arm's reach from heaven. At the top of Mount Lincoln (elevation 5,089 feet), I stopped for a rest break and a photo shoot, certain that sherpas and yaks would be following me.

Like a bizarre dream, my mountain ecstasy was short lived. A mile later on the top of Mount Lafayette, I found myself weaving my way through a horde of Japanese tourists armed with expensive cameras. On a bus tour, they had hiked to the peak from Greenleaf Hut. Frustrated, I hiked to Garfield Ridge Shelter to get far away from the maddening crowd.

Disappointed that I wasn't able to work-for-stay at the hut, I was thrilled to have the shelter to myself for at least a couple of hours. At dusk, two female overnight hikers in their early twenties arrived with 2 six-packs of Blue Moon ale. Of course, free beer and two lovely young ladies were guaranteed to draw a crowd, even on a wilderness mountaintop. Minutes later, the caretaker for the campground and a trail crew supervisor materialized from the shadows to inquire about our welfare, or more aptly their welfare.

A campfire was quickly started, and I spent two entertaining hours listening to adventures in the Whites from the interlopers while downing a couple of cold brews. I didn't know which was funnier, the story about the bear that was stealing bear boxes or the dismantled shelter that was helicoptered to the wrong mountain.

The next morning my "Blue Moon over the Mountain" euphoria dissipated within minutes after stepping on the trail. "This is insane. This is no trail," I shouted at the trees. I backtracked to make sure that I hadn't missed a turnoff. I hadn't. I peered over the edge of a small waterfall trying to figure out how I was going to reach the bottom without a rappelling rope or parachute.

Looking for an alternate route, I noticed a line of trees that had been stripped of bark and branches. Following that lead, I grabbed every branch within reach and lowered myself to the bottom. After a steep climb to South Twin Mountain, the wings fell completely off my backpack. My soaring spirit was grounded in another fog bank. All I could see were wood signs on the top of a rock maze that looked like the crosses at Calvary.

Emerging from an evergreen forest, I rock hopped on boulders toward Mount Guyot as a stout wind was blowing the fog off the mountaintops. In the distance, I could see and hear the rain moving toward me. I stopped and watched the visceral drama unfold. *Alone on the mountain, staring down a storm. That's the making of a real mountain man,* I thought before turning to the summit. Looking up, I saw a flash of movement in the rocks next to the trail. A mountain lion, bobcat, or Big Foot was my first thought. As I drew closer, the forms began to take shape. They weren't hikers but two young women with notebooks and measuring devices in their hands. Despite the approaching storm, I stopped to make their acquaintance out of scientific curiosity.

A few minutes later, David Taylor, a biology professor at the University of Portland in Oregon, joined us. He and his graduate students were conducting a survey of alpine vegetation. Because of its location on the East coast, the Whites were a living laboratory for studying weather, global warming, and pollution. Everything in the atmosphere from the West coast ended up in these mountains.

With the rain falling, I headed back up the trail. Near the top, I looked down and saw the group frantically waving at me with outstretched arms. Fearing I was in danger from a wild animal or a misstep, I spun around. Nothing! As I waved back, David raced toward me. I didn't dare take another step until I knew the emergency.

"I'm sorry. I gave you directions to the shelter, not the trail," he said apologetically while catching his breath. "You missed the turnoff. Follow me and I'll take you back."

About a half a mile from the Zealand Falls Hut, I encountered more maidens. This time it was three long and lean blondes somewhere in their late twenties or early thirties. Bounding up the trail in brightly colored Spandex shorts and tops, they were bubbling with enthusiasm and energy. Meanwhile, I was stumbling down the trail bone-tired with a long face after a hard day in the mountains. "Where are you coming from?" I asked anxiously, hoping that I was just steps from the hut.

"We're staying at the hut with our families. It's kind of a mountain vacation," one of the ladies replied before heading up the mountain. I watched them disappear in the trees, still shaking my head and blinking my eyes.

About twenty minutes later, I arrived at the hut with a sigh of relief. After registering for work-for-stay, I walked over to the falls to soak my tired and aching feet. Sitting next to me was a couple with a carton of wine and a handful of plastic cups. Doris and Ken were more than willing to share their libation with a mountain man.

"A march of the mountain maidens. After days of seeing nothing but ragtag hikers, they were a most welcomed sight, especially the last group in Spandex," I cheerfully proclaimed, replaying the day's events.

"Hair in ponytails?" Doris asked.

"Yep, then you saw them too," I replied.

"That's our daughters," Ken howled with laughter. About a half an hour later, daughters 1 (Sue), 3 (Janice), and 7 (Beth) as they were numerically named, joined us at the stream for a drink. With my feet in the water, a glass of wine in my hand, and a smile on my face, the ladies jokingly commented on my quick recovery.

Later that day, I met Utah, a gangly young man in his early twenties from the state of Utah. Since we were the only two hikers at the hut, we were warmly welcomed by the "croo." In return for sweeping the dining room floor and cleaning the bunkhouse, we dined on stuffed shells, chicken in wine sauce, and lasagna. Breakfast was oatmeal and pancakes with a couple strips of leftover bacon, a rarity in the huts. Being an early NOBO was already reaping rewards.

After saying good-bye to Ken, Doris, and the daughters, who generously made a donation to Herm's Hike, I headed down the trail to Crawford Notch, the gateway to Mount Washington. In the bright sunshine, I hiked a pleasant seven miles that included a scenic pond, a couple of boardwalks, a suspension bridge, and a generous section of old railroad bed. The only thing missing was the maidens.

Utah was waiting for me at Highland Center Lodge in Crawford Notch. With the promise of good weather on Mount Washington, the best to date, we hiked to Mizpah Spring Hut for another night of work-for-stay. We were officially in the Presidential Range. The tallest peak in the Northeast at 6,288 feet was calling.

The next morning under sunny skies, I began the six-mile ascent to Mount Washington alone. During a rest break at the Lakes of the Clouds Hut, I discovered that I had lost a water bottle. No need to panic with a well-stocked hiker's box. I merely exchanged my one for a matching pair. Trail karma was paying daily dividends.

The next mile and a half hike to the summit of Mount Washington was steep, rocky, and windy. By the time I reached the summit at around noon, the wind was blowing at 35 miles per hour with temperatures in the mid-50s. I was lucky to have such a balmy day. Bad weather was the norm for the crossroad of storm fronts from around the country. Temperatures above 60 degrees were rare, occurring a dozen times a year. On April 12, 1934, a record wind speed of 231 mph was recorded at the summit. On January 16, 2004, the record low temperature with wind chill was recorded at -102.5 degrees Fahrenheit.

The mountain was to be respected in all seasons. Weather conditions changed from idyllic to disastrous in seconds. Since 1849, nearly 150 people had lost their lives. Only a week earlier, a hiker had fallen to his death at Tuckerman Ravine. One of the more notable deaths on the memorial list in the main building belonged to William Buckingham Curtis. Considered the "father of American amateur sports," Curtis died from exhaustion and hypothermia near the Lakes of the Clouds Hut in a summer snowstorm on June 30, 1900. Mother Nature did not discriminate among the foolhardy.

Inside the building complex, I followed the excited mob of day tourists to the cafeteria where I feasted on pizza. After lunch, I took a few pictures at the summit sign before hitting the trail.

For a short distance, the trail followed the cog railway down the mountain. When the steam engine and passenger car appeared on its ascent, I stopped and waved, discarding the unsavory tradition of "mooning the cog." In 2007, undercover cops busted eight hikers after they dropped their pants, a federal offense on government property. Being a domestic terrorist was enough notoriety for me. I laughed aloud wondering if the Hole in the Wall Gang with Butch and Sundance had ever mooned the trains they robbed. That would have been a hilarious scene in the movie. I laughed ever harder when I realized the cog could have ended the war in Vietnam. I hilariously envisioned thousands of young men lined up along the rails with their pants down. Who would fight the war if all draft-eligible men were rejected for criminal convictions? Arlo could have penned another musical ode to our generation. The thin mountain air was making me giddy.

Descending to the bottom of Edmands Col, a drop of nearly 2,000 feet over three miles, rock cairns replaced white blazes. Instead of rock scrambling, I was boulder climbing and hopping, often descending on the seat of my pants.

At the bottom of the col, I noticed a lone hiker heading toward me. At first, I thought it was Utah, but as the solitary figure drew closer, I noticed he was much shorter and much older. When the hiker was within a few yards of me, I stopped and stepped aside. "Great day to be in the mountains," I greeted cheerfully. Without a word, the man glided by me as if I was invisible. A large floppy hat, pulled over his forehead, hid his face.

As the figure grew smaller, I stared at his unique gait. He moved with the mannerisms of my father. A chill ran down my spine. "Dad, is that you?" I hollered instinctively, but it was too late. The vaporous figure disappeared among the boulders, never to reappear on the ridge. "Just a day hiker," I muttered, trying to convince myself this chance encounter was nothing more than my frenzied imagination.

Later in the day, I caught up with Utah at Madison Spring Hut, home for the night. "Did you pass that old guy on the trail?" I asked nonchalantly.

"The only person I saw after lunch was you and that was from the other side of the mountain," he replied.

"Lot of trails up on the ridge. Probably, just another day hiker," I mumbled, still pondering the mysterious hiker.

At dinner, I finally witnessed a performance from the "croo." With songs and skits, it was improv comedy at its finest by college kids who weren't afraid to gore the sacred cows of the hiking world, to include thru-hikers and tree huggers. After a hot meal of leftovers, Utah and I washed dishes for about an hour. Before lights out, one of the croo offered me an open bunk at no charge. Old age along with karma was also paying dividends.

In the morning, I stayed late for a pancake breakfast while Utah headed out early for the next hut thirteen miles away. My destination was seven miles up the trail to Pinkham Notch where I hoped to find a room at the lodge. The only challenge of the day was Mount Madison, a climb of 1,500 feet in half a mile, just behind the hut. By early afternoon, I was standing in front of the reception desk at Joe Dodge Lodge. To my disappointment, there was no room at the inn. The lodge was booked for the next two days.

Outside, I ate lunch at one of the picnic tables, rested, and frowned. The next hut was six miles away after a steep climb up Wildcat Mountain. I would need all the energy that I could muster.

"Can I offer you some gorp?" a man asked kindly, carrying a box filled with bags of the trail snack.

"Thank you," I said, stashing it in my backpack. "But what I really need is a place to stay."

"If you can wait here for a few minutes. I'll give you a ride to Gorham."

A few minutes later, the gorp distributor reappeared behind the wheel of his car. My trail angel was trail legend Leon Barkman, who in 1967 became the thirty-seventh person to thru-hike the AT. A bona fide outdoorsman, he had also hiked the forty-nine highest peaks in the contiguous United States. Now in his early eighties, the retired biology teacher maintained his connection with the AT community with day hikes and slideshow presentations at the lodge. Personal friends of trail legends Earl Shaffer, Gene Espy (the second person to thru-hike the AT), and Grandma Gatewood, he was an AT pioneer who hiked before trail names became fashionable.

Leon dropped me off at the Barn, an old New England barn that had been converted to a spacious and comfortable hiker hostel. The next morning at 7 o'clock sharp, Leon was waiting at the curb for my ride back to the trail. I was sorry the ride wasn't longer. Leon was a walking almanac of trail knowledge and trail stories. I was thrilled to have met an AT original and legend. They were a vanishing species.

I bagged seven peaks in thirteen miles before stopping at the Imp Shelter for the evening. Earlier in the day, I stopped at the Carter Notch Hut, the last hut in the Whites, for a coffee and learned that I had missed Utah by a day. The next day I hiked over Mount Moriah and hitched a ride back to the Barn. With numerous rock climbs, the hiking was difficult. I was ready for a zero day.

Back at the hostel, I called home. Brite was gushing with her own amazing trail story. After posting my entry about Chet's Place, Brite's aunt from a nearby town in Maine called her to say that she used to babysit Chet and his brother. It was a small world and trail, after all.

After picking up my mail drop the following day, I explored the town and visited the railroad museum. That evening after dinner, I had a chance encounter with another legend. In the parking lot of a strip mall, I noticed a large blue and green globe next to a van. I walked over to investigate.

The man sitting on the bumper was Erik Bendl, famously known as the World Guy. Since 2007, he had been pushing his six-foot inflatable globe, named the

World, around the country to promote the American Diabetes Association. Along with his dog Nice, he had walked thousands of miles up and down the East coast and as far west as Pike's Peak. Tomorrow he was walking the auto road to Mount Washington with his globe. His inspiration was his mother, who died from the disease at the age of fifty-four.

After trading stories about fund raising, I reached in my pocket and pulled out a twenty-dollar bill as a donation.

"But what about Herm's Hike? Shouldn't this be going to the Alzheimer's Association?" Erik said apologetically.

"No, not this time. You just gave me the inspiration to finish a long and difficult journey. That's priceless," I replied earnestly.

Before leaving, I clumsily tried my hand at pushing the globe around the parking lot. It was like chasing a beach ball on a windy day. Like hiking the AT, "globing" was something easier said than done.

Early the next morning, fueled by a healthy dose of inspiration, a good night's sleep, and a pancake breakfast, I hit the trail alone. Two miles beyond Mount Success, I happily stood next to the boundary for Maine. I had finally reached the last state on the trail. There were only 281.8 miles to Mount Katahdin. Making my way down to Carlo Col Shelter for the night, a large rattlesnake was swallowing a large frog in the middle of the trail. With no place to safely step around rocks, I waited about five minutes before it slowly slithered away. Not one to believe in bad omens, I didn't construe the serpent as a nefarious omen.

Chapter 26

Finding a Bodhi Tree

(Carlo Col Shelter to Monson, ME)

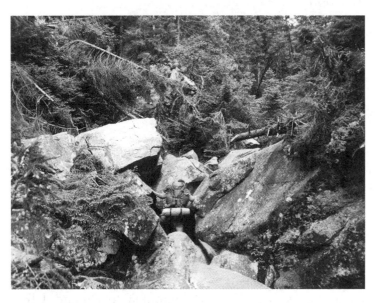

A hiker entering Mahoosuc Notch, the toughest mile on the trail.

Shortly after crossing the state line, I quickly realized that Maine's reputation as the toughest state on the trail was the undisputed truth. The hike to the summit of Goose Eye Mountain was a hand-over-hand climb with rebar steps and a series of wood ladders. It was like scaling a castle wall. One slip of a hand or foot and you could easily plunge to your death. I shuddered to think the toughest mile on the AT was just ahead, the Mahoosuc Notch Trail.

At Fulling Mill Mountain, I began the steep descent to the notch. Surprisingly, the trail wasn't a rock scramble, but there were plenty of twigs and stones on the ground that acted like ball bearings under my feet. I stepped deliberately, making sure my feet were firmly planted before taking the next step.

About halfway down, my left foot started to slowly slide forward after a slow and measured step. Afraid I was going to tumble forward, I leaned to my right on my hiking pole to break my fall. As I twisted in slow motion, I heard the crackle and crunch of ligaments in my left ankle. I landed on my right side with my left leg awkwardly pinned beneath my body. My left foot burned with pain.

"No, no, no! I don't believe this is happening," I screamed in agony as an expletive-laced tirade tumbled down the mountainside. Slowly I rolled over to free my leg. Using my hiking poles, I gradually rose to a standing position. A thick, greasy sweat trickled down my cheeks. Looking down with relief, I saw no protruding bones or red blotches. My concern now was the extent of any internal damage. Until I removed my boots, the only visible damage was a bowed hiking pole.

Catching my breath, I calmed down and realized the injury might not be that severe. This was my chronically weak ankle that I had rolled in Nantahala. Only this time, there was the sickening sound of crunching ligaments. That's what had me worried. I tightened my boot and stepped gingerly down the mountain. As long as I could tolerate the pain, I could move forward. I still had the toughest mile on the trail ahead of me.

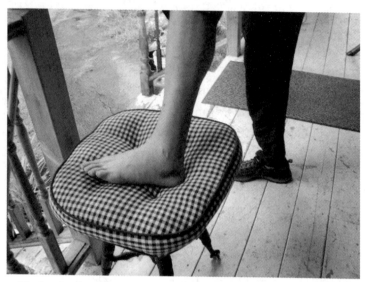

My damaged ankle after the Notch. Pain becomes synonymous with Maine.

The Mahoosuc Notch was a narrow gap in a walled canyon filled with large, jagged, and uneven boulders. It looked like a dumpsite for leftover debris after God created the mountains. For two hours, I painstakingly crawled, clawed, and climbed through nature's obstacle course. Every few feet, I had to stop and plan my next step. At times, I was forced to climb up the face of a boulder and leap to the next one. With a gimpy ankle, it was risky maneuver, but it had to be done. In some of the crevices, I had to remove my backpack and push it forward before squeezing through the opening.

After scrambling underneath the last boulders, I wiped the sweat from my face with a sigh of relief. The worst was over, but I was far from finished. Staring down at me was the second toughest mile on the trail. The Mashoosuc Arm was a rock climb and scramble that ascended 1,200 feet in just under a mile. Once again, I followed the line of broken branches to hoist myself up a few feet at a time. Stopping for frequent breaks, I realized that I was not alone. Attracted by my salty sweat, swarms of golden butterflies alighted on my arms and backpack. *If these tiny angels could only carry me up this mountain*, I thought wistfully.

Mercifully after reaching the top of the arm, Speck Pond Shelter was only a tortuous mile away. For the rest of the day, I soaked my ankle in the mountain pond. There was only slight swelling and no discoloration as of yet. Too tired to boil water for a hot meal, I had a dinner of Spam sandwiches and a healthy dose of Vitamin I.

"Think deeper. It's more than a spirit animal. It's a spiritual transformation, a rebirth," one of the female New Age hikers proclaimed after I told my butterfly story around the campfire.

"Kind of a painful way to start over," I joked.

"Most births are. Remember no pain, no gain, no Maine." She chuckled, reciting her impromptu version of AT mantra. It was certainly food for thought.

By 8 o'clock, I was in my sleeping bag sound asleep despite the throbbing ankle. The next morning after a breakfast of Pop Tarts and a healthy dose of ibuprofen, I hiked four miles down the mountain using my hiking poles as crutches. The ankle was considerably swollen, but I was able to painfully squeeze my foot into my boot.

At Grafton Notch, trail magic was two 16-ounce Rolling Rock beers and a ride halfway to the hostel in Andover. Still too far to walk, I stuck out my thumb and waited patiently on the lightly traveled country road. Ten minutes later, a menacing black pickup stopped. Muddy and battered with oversized tires, it looked as if it had been driven off the set of a Stephen King movie. In the passenger's seat was Phil the Bear Man, a barrel-chested outdoorsman who worked as a hunting guide.

"If you don't mind a little detour, I can give you a ride into town. Don't want to sit in the back, though. Nothing but blood and guts," Phil joked as he scooted to the center. Only Phil wasn't joking. In the bed of the truck were twenty 5-gallon plastic buckets of offal. Phil was on his way to bait his bear stations somewhere in the wilds of Maine, and I was along for the ride. Behind the wheel was a young woman who I thought was his teenage bride. It turned out to be Phil's daughter who had just received her learner's permit.

A likely story to lure me into the woods and dismember me, I thought. Crazy thoughts swirled through my head. No one would ever find my body after the bears had finished with me. A few minutes later, we stopped at a steel gate just off the road with a No Trespassing sign. Worriedly, I watched Phil open, close, and lock the gate behind us. Picturing in my mind a Maine version of the movie *Deliverance*, I was ready to bolt from the truck and flag down the next car. With my luck, it would have been Phil's brother or cousin.

Bouncing along the rutted road, Phil launched into his monologue about the perils of bear hunting. More worry. After four bait stops that took us deep into the woods, we finally turned around. As Phil drove me to the Pine Ellis Hostel, I realized that he was just a teddy bear in disguise. While he wasn't the inspiration for a Stephen

King character, one thing was certain. If you ever wanted to get rid of a body, there was no better place than a bait station in the backwoods of Maine.

I holed up at the hostel for two nights to rehab the ankle. On the front porch, I propped up my ankle and applied a frozen bag of peas on the hour. The ankle and foot had ballooned and turned a sickly yellowish hue with streaks of blue and purple. No longer able to squeeze my foot into the boot, I hobbled around in my camp shoes. It wasn't as painful as it looked, but it generated sympathy from my fellow hikers.

After two days of rest, I gingerly squeezed my foot into my boot and slackpacked ten miles from Grafton Notch back to Andover with only minor discomfort. The test run went so well that I decided to slackpack the thirty-five miles to Rangeley. Searching for a hiking partner, I looked no further than Squeezecheese, another lame hiker convalescing at the hostel. With his knees wrapped in Ace bandages like a mummy, he wasn't sure if he could take another step on the trail. With 260 miles to go, he was determined to finish no matter what it took.

During my stay, he continually queried hikers about slackpacking to Rangeley. There were no takers. Now after my test run, I jumped at the chance. Two days later with light daypacks and lighter wallets, we hiked triumphantly into Rangeley. My foot was still discolored and stiff, but I was hiking with no pain. The only disturbing issue was a grotesque, large knot on the back of my left leg.

At the Gull Pond hostel in Rangeley, a hiking nurse said that I might have a stress fracture or muscle tear. She strongly recommended I have the foot X-rayed. I called

Brite for her opinion and she agreed wholeheartedly.

The next day while Squeezecheese hit the trail, Bob O'Brien, the hostel owner, drove me to a clinic in Farmington with an X-ray machine. There were no breaks or fractures, and the diagnosis was second-degree ankle sprain with a tear/rupture of the plantaris tendon, which explained the lump on the back of my leg. The tendon, dating back to when man first starting walking upright, was a superficial muscle used primarily for transplants. As long as I wasn't in pain, the doctor saw no reason why I couldn't hike. They recommended that I purchase an elastic ankle brace. Just another one added to the collection back home.

Later that afternoon, Bob picked me up with grim news. After dropping me off, he took his ailing dog, a beautiful Labrador, to the veterinarian. Cancerous tumors had spread throughout her body. Her hair had fallen out in clumps, and her hind legs were paralyzed. The humane option was to put her to sleep.

Checking out the next day, I offered to pay for the ride to Farmington, but Bob wouldn't take my money. "I was headed there anyway, plus I had some company. Make that some good company, so maybe I should pay you," he joked.

At the trailhead, I asked Bob if he needed more "good company" for the ride to the vet's. He was headed back to say a final good-bye to his beloved Gwendy. "I think I need some time alone. We've been together fourteen years. Old dogs and old men have a lot in common," he replied sadly. I simply nodded in agreement.

Armed with a favorable medical diagnosis, or as good as it was going to get for the rest of the hike, and an elastic ankle brace, I was excited to tackle the last big mountain ranges in Maine. From Rangeley to Stratton, I climbed four mountains over 4,000 feet. On the first day, I hiked from Saddleback Mountain to Saddleback Junior over the mountain spine above the tree line. It looked and felt like the Whites.

Mountains rolled to the horizon while below hundreds of ponds glistened in the sunlight like diamonds. With no roads, buildings, or ski resorts in sight, I was seeing the wilderness that captured the literary rapture of Uncle Hank. Thoreau found these mountains to be a transcendent experience, a reflection of his relationship with the cosmos. I was soon to discover how transcendent the mountains could be.

In the late afternoon, I arrived at the Poplar Ridge Lean-To (a shelter was a lean-to in Maine). Although I had hiked only eleven miles, it had been a satisfying day. With the ankle still tender, there was no need to push big mile days. A couple of hikers stopped briefly for a rest break before heading up the trail. That night I had the shelter to myself.

After dinner, I read from my Thoreau book before darkness settled. With my bed already prepared, I sat on the edge of the shelter entrance in a yoga position with my hands resting on my knees and my index fingers and thumbs forming small circles. It was an unconscious yet natural position that relaxed my body. I sat for over an hour in total silence and watched the woods fade to an impenetrable black. Cloaked in total darkness, I gently closed my eyes and fell into a meditative state. My ears heard only silence of the night. My mind heard only the silence of the soul. Any intruding thoughts had been stilled. Slowly, I felt my body become a tingling entity, alive and awake, floating in a pool of tranquility as if I were floating in heaven.

As images of the day seeped back into my brain, I slowly opened my eyes. Hoping not to break the mystical spell with light from my headlamp, I crawled in the darkness to my sleeping bag. Closing my eyes, a tidal wave of thoughts flooded my brain. My first thought was about Bob. I hoped he was safely home, asleep in a rocker with a picture of Gwendy in his lap. I hoped his assistant Bonnie was gazing at the stars and remembering her deceased husband with a soft smile. I hoped Edward, the resident wannabe hiker, was checking his backpack one last time before heading out for the trail in the morning.

Before drifting off to sleep, I opened my eyes and searched the night sky. The universe of endless bright lights in the heavens had been created from nothing, a vacuum of silent darkness that reached to infinity. At my birth, I had passed through the darkness into the light of the world, and one day would pass again through the darkness into the light of the universe. With divine light, we saw the beauty of humanity through our eyes. With divine darkness, we saw the beauty of the soul through God's illuminating eyes.

"Sondance, your brain is going to explode trying to decipher the mysteries of the universe," I chuckled before closing my eyes. Focusing on my breathing with shallow and slow breaths, pictures of mountain vistas from Georgia to Maine flashed underneath my eyelids like a slide show. Peacefully I fell asleep before the show ended, hopefully to be continued at a later date.

Later that night I had a visitor. I was walking

along a ridgeline when I saw him about fifty yards ahead of me. He moved haltingly. I quickened my pace. Drawing closer, I recognized the silhouette as the man that I saw hiking in the col to Mount Washington. Only this time, he was wearing a blue headband similar to mine.

I started to run faster, but frustratingly fell farther behind with each step. My boots were sinking into the mountain. Sweat stung my eyes. I screamed in anguish but no words came from my mouth. Just before the man stepped down the mountain, he stopped and faced me. My body shuddered. I bolted upright in my sleeping bag. "Dad," I shouted into the darkness. The face belonged to a twenty-year-old private first class stationed at Schofield Barracks, Hawaii, in 1941.

I wiped the cold sweat from my face and sank back into the warm caress of my sleeping bag. Unlike many other dreams that were bizarre snippets of the subconscious, this one was so life-like that I wanted to see how it ended. Minutes later, after my mind had relaxed, I fell into a deep, dreamless sleep. That night the shelter had become my Bodhi Tree. A ray of enlightenment, merely a flicker of spiritual light, had burned through the darkness and touched my soul.

The next morning I was up with the sun ready to tackle the next mountain range. As I shouldered my backpack, I reached for the blue headband in my pants pocket. It wasn't there or anywhere around the shelter. I finally found it on the trail in front of the shelter where I had obviously dropped it. I wondered what I would do if I found a second one farther up the trail.

After nearly sixty miles of breathtaking mountain ridges and a hostel stop in Stratton, I reached the

Kennebec River, another major milestone on the trail. Still early in the morning, I waited about an hour for the ferryman Hillbilly Dave to arrive. The ferry was a sixteen-foot canoe that carried hikers across a dangerous stretch of river. With a hydroelectric dam upriver that released water for rafters and kayakers, water levels could rise two to four feet within seconds. In 1985, a hiker got caught in a surge while trying to ford the river and was washed downriver to her death.

After signing my release form, I climbed into the canoe with the white blaze on the bottom. Five minutes later I set foot on solid ground and was rewarded with a cooler filled with sodas, beer, candy bars, and cookies. I hiked through the Maine woods on a sugar high.

A few miles south of Moxie Pond, I met an elderly gentleman out for a day hike. "My truck is back at the pond. If you want a ride into town, just wait for me. I'll be there in about an hour."

I decided to take him up on his offer. While waiting at the pond, a young family invited me to join their picnic. In exchange for tales from the trail, I received a lunch of fried chicken and potato salad. I could still yogi with the best of them.

As promised, Peter returned about an hour later. The twelve-mile ride to town on the old logging road that followed the old railroad bed took just under two hours, but I didn't mind a bit. Along the way, Peter provided a running narration of life in Bingham, the Canada Road, and the Somerset Railway. He also promised a place to stay.

Peter dropped me off at the Eagle's Nest, a rental house primarily used for hunters and snowmobilers. For

$30, I had a three-bedroom house with kitchen, full bath, and living room with a television. That evening Mike, the next-door neighbor, brought me a plate of meat loaf, green beans, and mashed potatoes.

"How long did it take to get here?" he laughed. In his own meticulous and methodical way, Peter had become a town legend. The next morning after breakfast with Mike and his family, Peter was at the back door at 8 a.m. sharp for the two-hour ride back to Moxie Pond. Obviously, I had more to learn about the history of Bingham, Maine.

Two days and two fords of the Piscataquis River later, I stepped onto Maine 15 and hitched a ride into Monson. My original plan was to stop in Monson and wait for Brite so we could hike the last one hundred miles together, but I was ahead of schedule. Feeling young and restless, meaning I was in peak hiking condition, I decided to spend the night in town at Shaw's Lodge, resupply, and head back to the trail. I wanted to finish at least half of the Wilderness before Brite arrived.

My main concern for the remaining miles was Brite. Maine had been more rugged than anticipated, and Brite didn't have a lot of time to train for the hike. When I had called her from Shaw's to finalize our meeting plans, she readily agreed that forty-six miles to Katahdin sounded better than one hundred and fourteen.

Back on the trail after Shaw's famous AYCE "one plate at a time" breakfast of eggs, bacon, sausage, and hash browns, I finally faced the famous Wilderness sign. It warned hikers to pack at least ten days of provisions, but since I was only going sixty miles, I traveled much lighter. The hyperbole about this section of the trail was not its difficulty but isolation. Except for a few logging roads and one hostel, this was a true wilderness.

The hiking was similar to traversing southern Appalachia, only this section had an abundance of Christmas trees, blueberries, and lakes. I fell in love with the lakes, taking a plunge whenever possible. After each wilderness baptism, I emerged from the cool water mentally and physically invigorated, ready to hike more miles.

On the trail, I counted down the miles and mountains. Between Monson and my stopping point at White House Landing, I climbed ten of the eleven mountain peaks to Mount Katahdin. At White Cap Mountain, the last big peak with an elevation of 3,650 feet, I had my first prolific view of Mount Katahdin. It rose from the valley floor like a dormant volcano, floating on an ivory sea of low clouds. "At long last, the finish line," I whispered triumphantly. There were only seventy-two miles to the summit.

On the fifth day of my expedition, I stood on the dock across from White House Landing and sounded the air horn. Fifteen minutes later, a runabout arrived and ferried me across Pemadumcook Lake. The camp was a little pricey but worth every penny. I ignored the comments from hikers about price gouging. After all, this was a wilderness outpost. For just over a hundred bucks, I had dinner (the famous one-pound hamburger), a bunk, breakfast, and a shuttle to Monson the following morning. At noon the following day, I was back at Shaw's Lodge with an indelible smile. My sweetheart was only two days away. Within a week, we would be heading home.

Chapter 27

An Apostle in Monson

(Monson to Millinocket, ME)

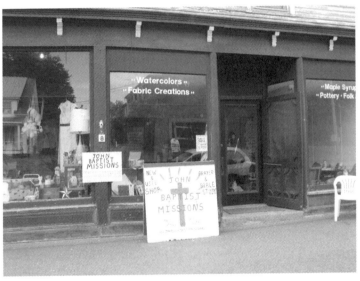

A spiritual outpost in Monson where Christ would feel at home.

Back in Monson, I quickly acquired the moniker of "The Mayor" from my fellow hikers. When walking the streets, adults and children called out my name and waved. I didn't tell my mystified hiking brethren that I had already visited the library, the fire department, and every restaurant, store, and church within sight.

On my first urban excursion, I stumbled upon the Swedish Lutheran Church. Built by the Swedish community in 1890, the ornate structure with brown clapboard siding, converted to offices, was now the home of the Areopagus II America Institute, a ministry of Christian apologetics. I had no idea about the group, but there was a welcome sign for hikers. I was hoping for a cup of coffee and a doughnut.

From around the corner appeared a wheelchair and the Reverend Daryl Witmer, founder of the institute who was felled by Guillain-Barre Syndrome in 1984. After a cordial greeting, Daryl led me to a display table with literature. There was no coffee or doughnuts, only heavy doses of evangelical interpretation. I quickly learned the apologetics were defenders of the Christian faith through the Bible.

"Are you a Christian?" Daryl asked politely.

"Old altar boy," I chuckled. Sensing this was going to be an evangelical litmus test, I tried to inject some humor into the conversation. From the dour look on his face, I saw that Daryl was not impressed with my answer.

"Do you believe the Bible is the word of God?"

"Right now, I believe the Bible is the word about God. It's a book filled with great wisdom and truth, but it's been written and rewritten and interpreted and misinterpreted. No one is really sure who wrote it or when it was written. To me, it's a guidebook that provides directions for the spiritual voyager," I responded. Daryl looked stunned as if I had just sprouted horns and a tail.

Any second, I expected to be pummeled with a cannonade of Bibles. To Daryl and his fellow apologetics, the only path to the summit of salvation was through Jesus Christ and Scripture exclusively. Muslims, Buddhists, Hindus, Druids, and the Twelve Tribes of Israel needn't queue at the pearly gates. Following that line of thinking, every religious conundrum, enigma, or other unexplainable event that defined their version of Christianity was simply answered with "the Bible says it's so."

We chatted a little longer, but I could see that Daryl was not interested in my spiritual journey. Likewise, I wasn't enamored with his defense of Christianity by spouting Bible verses. I found his explanations theological doublespeak. Word games for the sake of scholarly argument were rhetorical gibberish.

I explained that spirituality is a personal experience and not the belief in someone else's experience. It must come from the heart and not the head. Mainstream religions can't accept the mystery of God without trying to explain everything that can't be explained. They are selling salvation by their book, and if you don't buy what they're selling, you'll never see the face of God. To me that was nonsense.

In the end, we politely agreed to disagree. I had no doubt Daryl dismissed me as a New Age religious kook who should be burned at the stake. Fearing a religious anxiety attack, I thanked Daryl for his time and quickly headed out the door. *If only the Eagle Man could have heard me. If only he had been standing by my side, the conversation would have made theological history,* I thought as I walked up the street to explore more of Monson. Little did I know that salvation was literally just around the corner.

Much to my surprise, the essence of Christianity

was found a block away at John Baptist Missions, a storefront thrift shop and Bible study/prayer center founded by Bettinan Stevens, simply known as Bett. Unlike the apologetics, there was no professionally painted sign attached to the building. An A-frame, wooden sign with hand-painted letters stood outside a dilapidated building. Inside were tables and shelves of donated clothing, appliances, housewares, sporting goods, baby items, and books. Everything was free. Donations were graciously accepted. While browsing for that buried treasure, I chatted with the effervescent Bett and made a donation for a couple of books.

Later that afternoon at Bett's invitation, I returned for a good cup of coffee (I brought the doughnuts) and a great conversation. While attending a prayer service in a last-ditch effort to battle her personal demons of addiction and abuse, she heard a loud and clear voice telling her to follow in the footsteps of Christ. That path eventually led her to establish a ministry in Monson. Bett leaned heavily on the Bible as her spiritual foundation, but, unlike the apologetics, her approach was casual and low-key. She noted that she frequently clashed with Daryl over Scripture and their ministries. Not surprisingly, he viewed her as a religious charlatan. She viewed him as a theological snob.

Bett listened in earnest as I described my encounters with Baptists, Buddhists, Brother Pius, and my guardian angels. I had no doubt that if Jesus Christ ever visited Monson, you would find him at the mission having a cup of coffee with Bett, one of his true apostles. The storefront would be a church that he recognized as home.

The following morning while waiting for Brite, I stopped at the mission to say good-bye and thank Bett for her hospitality with a cash donation.

"Wait right here, I have something for you," she announced cheerfully, walking to the back of the store. She quickly returned and handed me a small package. I looked at the wrapping and laughed politely.

"But it's not my birthday," I exclaimed.

"When you're born again, every day could be your birthday. Besides, it's all I could find," she smiled.

I tore away the paper and stared teary eyed at my gift, a book titled *Fathers Playing Catch with Sons (Essays on Sport Mostly Baseball)*. After the word "Sons," Bett had attached a yellow sticker that said, "and daughters." Obviously, Bett was listening when I told her that I regretted never having that final game of catch with my dad. In its place, I relished the memory when my daughter and I played catch in our yard at World Series time. There was always unspoken magic, actually unspoken love, in the air on those autumn afternoons. I wished that I could have given Bett a blank check.

While walking up the hill to the hostel, a woman was walking down the street and waving at me. It was Gram Cracker from last year's hike.

"Your women are waiting for you. Your wife just pulled into Shaw's, and Rockamimi just walked into town. Don't leave until she gets back. She wants to speak with you," she announced happily. In the hostel's parking lot, Brite greeted me with a long-awaited hug and a kiss. In return, I breathed a huge sigh of relief.

Her arrival singled the final leg of Herm's Hike. I had been worrying about her since she hit the road two days ago. From Parkton to Monson, it's just over six hundred fifty miles with the last forty miles along the back roads of the Maine wilderness. It's a long drive for anyone not familiar with the area. It's a longer drive for a woman traveling by herself.

Rockamimi returned shortly with a beaming smile. She had followed my trail journal and sent me a consoling e-mail after my father's death. Now she was hiking with Gram Cracker, who was finishing the last section of her AT hike.

"Are you still hiking to raise money for Alzheimer's?" she asked.

"Rather passively to be honest. I raised about eight hundred dollars since Vermont, but the real reason I came back was to finish the hike and place my memorial on top of Katahdin," I replied excitedly, quickly retelling the story of the sacred rock.

When Brite retrieved the rock and handed it to her, tears streamed down her cheeks. Everyone stood in stunned silence. I didn't understand the emotional outburst until I looked at the rock. Underneath the Herm's Hike logo were the names of Alzheimer's loved ones. Her father's name was the first on the list.

Wiping the tears from her eyes, she hugged me tightly. "Sondance, I can never thank you enough for remembering my father this way. I will never forget you as long as I live," she whispered hoarsely.

Brite and I climbed into our vehicle with tears in our eyes. I would never forget Rockamimi either. The time we spent talking about our fathers was an emotional highlight forever etched in my memory.

Heading down the road to Millinocket, I looked

over at Brite. "In a way, it's a shame that we're almost at the trail's end. There is always another good story waiting to be found," I said wistfully. Brite nodded her head in agreement about finding more stories, certainly not about hiking more miles. Little did I know at the time, the trail and the stories never end.

In town, we rendezvoused with Jamie, our shuttle driver and owner of the AT Lodge and AT Café with her husband, Paul. Noticing the magnet signs on the doors of the SUV, she asked about Herm's Hike; namely, who was Herm? I told her about my father and a little about his WWII combat experience. Farther down the road, she asked how Brite and I met.

"I was a navy nurse and Paul was a Marine Corps officer at Camp Pendleton, California. We were living in the BOQ (bachelor officer quarters) but didn't meet until introduced by a mutual friend who was in Paul's unit," Brite explained.

"My husband, Paul, was also a marine," Jamie chortled. What followed was one of the most compelling and heroic tales from the trail.

In 1971, while on patrol in Vietnam, Paul stepped on a landmine and was medevaced by helicopter to a field hospital. The force of the explosion shattered his femur, ripping apart muscle and bone. In a superhuman effort to save the leg, the surgeon inserted a metal rod. Although Paul kept the leg, he had to endure countless additional surgeries and therapy to restore as much mobility as possible.

In 2001, while on his first thru-hike attempt, he fell and broke his surgically repaired leg in the Smokies. This time he was medevaced by helicopter to a hospital in Ashville for surgery. After the operation, the surgeon asked Jamie if Paul had sustained his injury in Vietnam. When she replied yes, he told her that he was the surgeon who had operated on Paul. The story had a happy ending in 2007 when Paul finally completed the AT as a section-hiker. Back at the lodge, I had noticed a man with a heavily scarred and gnarled leg who walked with an odd gait like my father. That was Paul.

Brite and I arrived at White House Landing in the early afternoon. Anxious to hit the trail, and even more anxious to complete the journey, we grabbed the first boat ride across the lake. At the first white blaze, we stopped for a selfie with wide grins. We were finally back on the trail together. Our thoughts raced back to our first day at Springer Mountain. True to form, our hike in Maine mirrored our first days in Georgia.

We hiked eight miles to the Wadleigh Stream Lean-To, spending the night with an eclectic group of hikers. Early the next morning, we hiked to the summit of Nesuntabunt Mountain for our first close-up view of Mount Katahdin. We stood spellbound. The fabled mountain was only thirty-six miles away.

Instead of stopping at the next shelter, which would have been another eight-mile day, we pushed onward another three miles to the Rainbow Spring Campsite. As in Georgia, we couldn't out hike the weather. At the campground, we huddled together under a thick canopy of tree branches and watched the raindrops. With a break in the storm, we scrambled madly to set up the tent. Once snuggly and safely inside, it started to pour.

"Welcome to Georgia," Brite joked sarcastically as we listened to the rain.

"Déjà vu, all over again," I replied wearily, glad that we weren't camped on a mountainside next to a stream.

The next day we broke camp at sunrise under clear skies, a rare event in Brite's AT history. With little time to train, Brite was silently struggling. Although this section was deemed to be the easiest in Maine, any mile in Maine was challenging. For our twelve-mile jaunt, we hiked at a leisurely pace with plenty of rest breaks. With the miles slowly evaporating, it was time to savor these last miles on the trail together and look for a moose that we never found.

In mid-afternoon, we stepped on Golden Road, an appropriately named logging road that served as the main thoroughfare in the region. After crossing Abol Bridge with its postcard view of Mount Katahdin, we stopped for the night at the Abol Bridge Campground. Opting for a room with a view of the great mountain, we splurged for a campsite along the river. That evening we celebrated with our last freeze-dried meal on the trail. As we ate, we watched the mountain slowly vanish in the shadows. Mother Nature was a magician extraordinaire.

The next morning after a junk food breakfast at the camp store, we headed out for a ten-mile hike to the Katahdin Stream Campground in Baxter State Park. Fueled by coffee, doughnuts, and candy bars, we reached the campground in the early afternoon for a shuttle ride into Millinocket to retrieve our vehicle.

While checking in at the front desk of the Katahdin Inn and Suites, we bumped into a familiar face that appeared from around the corner. Brite and I stopped dead in our tracks with widening smiles. Flatlander had summited the mountain the previous day and was heading home. We had last seen him at Trail Days last year. The trail had come full circle.

Chapter 28
Climb(ed) Every Mountain
(Baxter State Park)

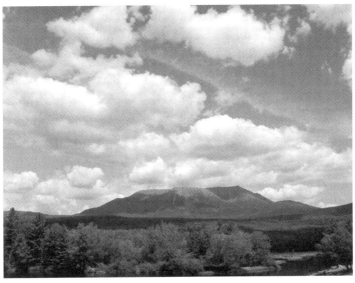

Brite and I enjoyed a stunning view of Mount Katahdin from our last campsite.

Back in Millinocket, Brite and I stopped by the Appalachian Trail Cafe for an early dinner. Sitting at one of the tables was Squeezecheese.

"Hiked up Katahdin yet?" he asked anxiously.

"Heading out first thing tomorrow morning and then heading home," I replied.

"Have room for one more?" he asked hopefully.

"If I didn't, I'd tie you to the luggage rack," I joked. "It would be an honor to finish the hike with you." Plus, I was glad to have an experienced hiker with us.

That night with the last mountain so close, I was too excited to sleep. All I could think about was finally touching the sign at the top of the legendary mountain with Brite by my side. That had been the dream since Springer Mountain.

The next morning, Brite and I headed out at 6 o'clock to pick up Squeezecheese. He was nervously pacing the sidewalk in front of the AT Café, just as anxious as we were about today's hike.

To guarantee entrance to Baxter State Park, I had reserved a parking space at Katahdin Stream Campground for Wednesday morning. When we stopped at the park entrance to register, the attendant spotted the Herm's Hike signs on the side of the SUV, asked a couple of questions about the hike, and then waived the $14 entrance fee. We were already riding a wave of good karma that I hoped would last through the day.

At the campground, we loaded our daypacks with cameras, Gatorade, snacks, sandwiches, and some foul weather gear. After registering at the ranger station and signing in at the trailhead, we headed up Hunt Trail. The weatherman was calling for a clear day and sunny skies with a high temperature near 80 (minimum of 15 degrees cooler on the mountain) and winds at 5 to 10 mph. Mother Nature was finally rewarding me for all of those windy and wet days.

For the first mile, the hike was a leisurely walk through a mixed pine forest. An alarm immediately sounded in my head. My trail book reported the 5.3-mile hike from campground to summit with an elevation gain of 4,188 feet. Throw out the first mile and that left an elevation gain of 4,188 over 4.3 miles. As the numbers danced crazily in my head, I thought about the difficulty in hiking in and out of Mahoosuc Notch. Not wanting to spook Brite, I kept my calculations to myself.

After reaching Katahdin Falls, we started to climb. First, it was a series of rock steps above the waterfalls and then rock outcroppings about every ten yards. With every step, the rocks got larger and the mountain steeper. The hike had become strictly a climb. Brite and I threw our hiking poles ahead of us, climbed hand over hand with the aid of a nearby tree branch, and retrieved our poles. We soon reached the point where the poles were collapsed and stuffed in the daypacks.

Progress was slow but steady until we reached the Gateway, an eight-foot rock wall with a rebar handle at the top. After several attempts, Brite couldn't grab the steel bar. Squeezecheese and I lifted her on our shoulders, but she still couldn't pull herself up and over the ledge.

"Guys, you go ahead and I'll wait here," she frowned, fearing the climb would be more difficult once we started scaling the spine of the mountain.

"If that's the case, then I'll stay with you and give the rock to Squeezecheese," I replied. Safety had been paramount since our first step at Springer Mountain. Now it was even more important, considering the remoteness of our location. Besides, there was no way I was going to leave my hiking partner of thirty years on the side of a mountain. And we were literally on the side of the mountain, huddled in a rocky nest high above the tree line with dizzying views of the surrounding mountains.

"I've got food, water, rain gear. If anything, I'm worried about you. Besides, it was never my hike. It was about you and your father. You carried his memory for over two thousand miles. You have to carry it for one more," Brite intoned firmly. I couldn't argue with her reasoning.

After Brite promised not to climb down the mountain by herself, Squeezecheese and I continued our climb. We quickly realized that leaving Brite behind was the right decision. Despite that reassuring thought, I felt as if I had abandoned her. I followed Squeezecheese with a sick feeling in the pit of my stomach.

After an hour of strenuous climbing, we crested the spine and laid eyes on the mountain plateau. We had reached the Tableland, a rocky dirt trail through a boulder-strewn, grassy slope. The summit of Katahdin was a mile ahead.

I cheered as Squeezecheese caught sight of the finish and raced ahead. Although anxious to join him, I still had one more stop. It was time to pay tribute to Uncle Hank, who despite his forays into the Maine wilderness never made it to the top of the mountain. At Thoreau Spring, I dipped my hand into the small pool only a few inches deep and pressed the holy water to my lips. With my spirit now purified, I was ready to take those final steps to the altar.

About half an hour later, I joined Squeezecheese on the top of Mount Katahdin. Named by the Penobscot Indians, it was the state's highest mountain at 5,267 feet. Today the "Greatest Mountain" was living up to its name in more ways than one. Ceremoniously, I walked up to the summit sign and kissed it. I had taken my last of five million steps. Herm's Hike was officially over.

Emotionally numb, I rested my hands on the top of the sign and gazed spellbound at the majestic view. Today I was AT royalty and wore the crown as "King of the Mountain." Below me, the glistening mountains and shimmering lakes knelt before me, bestowing their beauty and serenity for my coronation. Tears streamed down my face as I remembered the miles and the memories.

Regaining my composure, I took the mandatory pictures in front, behind, and on top of the sign. Stepping back from the sign, I opened my daypack, gently lifted the memorial rock, and placed it beneath the sign. In the bright sunshine, it sparkled like a diamond. Brite had painted the rock white and then hand-painted the logos for Herm's Hike and the Alzheimer's Association with the names of Alzheimer's victims. As instructed by Red Feather, I also placed prayer bundles of tobacco and sage under the sign, signifying the four directions and the cycle of life.

Hikers gathered around as I explained the history of the rock. They watched intently as I moved around the summit to complete the ritual of thankfulness. In a nearby cairn, I placed a memorial card with the names of all the Alzheimer's families that I encountered on the hike. In a rock crevice, I placed the remaining green tags with Justin's poems.

As I walked away, my fellow hikers began to gently clap. Teary eyed, I turned around for one final look at the summit and saluted my AT family. Squeezecheese and I bounded down the mountain with tattooed smiles, passing a number of hikers headed to the top.

"Have you seen the hiker at the Gate?" I inquired worriedly.

"Oh, so you're the guy who left his wife on the side of the mountain," a few hikers playfully chided while reassuring me that Brite was alive and in good spirits. Everyone on the way to the summit had met "Cathy Katahdin" as she was affectionately named by a hiker.

For over two hours, Brite had been greeting, meeting, cajoling, and cheering hikers to the summit with a contagious smile while waiting for her husband to return. At her trail's end, she proved to be the epitome of the AT hiker, whether it be a thru-hiker, a section hiker, a one-day hiker, a one-hour, or a one-step hiker. Her hike like mine had been a journey not a destination. She had hiked her own hike in her inimitable style. She and Uncle Hank had a lot in common.

Triumphantly leaving the Gate, we literally slid down the mountain on the seat of our pants and arrived at the parking lot nine hours after we had left. We immediately headed to the AT Café for a victory dinner and few victory beers to toast our success. Before leaving the cafe, we signed the traditional ceiling panel for the AT Class of 2010. After dropping off an exhausted and jubilant Squeezecheese at the AT Lodge, Brite and I headed back to the inn for the night.

Tomorrow we were headed home to start our official retirement. I could only wonder where that journey would take us. Although not a die-hard Grateful Dead fan, I fell asleep with the lyrics from their song "Truckin'" playing in my head: "Lately it occurs to me, What a long strange trip it's been." I had lived that lyric many times on the trail.

Chapter 29

Wednesdays with Frannie

(Parkton, MD)

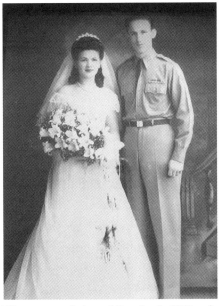

Frances and Herman on their wedding day in 1945, a love story that flourished for sixty-four years.

Sitting in front of my computer, at home, I savored the e-mails from my trail journal followers with a sense of elation instead of last year's utter frustration. One congratulatory note that delighted Brite and myself was from Wayne, a fellow marine and dear friend, who introduced us at Camp Pendleton. He often boasted about his matchmaking skills and rightfully so. Thirty-three years ago, none of us could have imagined that a brief introduction would eventually lead to the altar and then the Appalachian Trail.

With my final journal entry, donations surged briefly before I closed the website page. The final total was just over $7,000, a gratifying number for a grassroots movement that operated mostly on word of mouth. On my Facebook page, I updated my religious views with "Transcendnaturism: Enhancing your relationship with God through the divinity of nature." That summed up the hike in one sentence. My transcendentalist uncles would have nodded in agreement.

Now officially retired from work and the trail, I chauffeured my mother to the nursing home where she continued her mission of mercy. Whenever she questioned the impact of her presence, I reminded her about B from the trail. "You're just being you in a state of being alive for others. Just being there, wherever there is, is enough," I playfully scolded her. "You're a light that reaches into the darkest corners of the nursing home." My mother always smiled at that last comment.

A year later my mother's own health problems finally caught up with her. She was slowly dying from multiple myeloma. Needing full-time care, she reluctantly moved in with my sister. Now it was time to sell the house. Being the only retired sibling, the unenviable task fell to me.

A week before closing on the sale, my mother gave away the furniture, rugs, appliances, and whatever could be carried out the door to family members. Now one day before handing over the keys to the new owners, I was standing in the empty family room as scenes from bygone holidays, baptisms, birthdays, anniversaries, danced around me in mirth and merriment. Gazing around the room with the exit of the last ghost, I realized that I had inherited my father's book collection by default. The bookshelves next to the fireplace had not been emptied. I grabbed some empty boxes.

The collection consisted of sixty-four books, mostly Civil War and WWII histories and biographies. The religious titles included biographies of his heroes and heroines, Saint Francis, Mother Teresa, Mother Collette (founder of the Franciscan Sisters of Saint Joseph), Thomas Merton, Bishop Fulton Sheen, and Pope John Paul II. There were also two Bibles with annotated margins and two books on Catholicism by Pope John Paul II that were bookmarked. The dog-eared books by the pope attracted my attention. I snatched them from the stack and found a comfortable spot on the floor.

A task that should have taken five minutes lasted an hour as I read through my father's eyes. In *Crossing the Threshold of Hope*, the essay "Buddha?" had been marked by a Franciscan prayer card titled "To Be Happy." In *Prayers and Devotions*, the essays "Walking toward God" and "Walking in God's Gaze" had been marked with postcards of the pope. On the last page of that book, my father had written the quote from Ralph Waldo Emerson: "All I have seen teaches me to trust The Creator for all I have not seen."

I sat with the book frozen in my hand feeling numb, stunned at the breadth of my father's spiritual journey. Was my father exploring Buddhism like Merton?

Was my father exploring the Transcendentalists like I had done? Was my father becoming a "cafeteria Catholic" like myself, plucking the finest concepts of other religions and incorporating them into his own theology? The parallels between our spiritual journeys were startling. Uncle Ralph's quote had summarized my spiritual transformation on the trail, yet there was no way that my father in his medical condition knew that I was hiking the AT. *Father like son or son like father*, I thought. Back home, I placed those two books in a prominent spot in my personal bookcase. I had found two more gold nuggets or two connecting dots.

With my mother now living with my sister, there was a change in schedules for my mother and me. Our special day moved from Saturday to Wednesday. Author Mitch Albom had Tuesdays with Morrie, which became the title of his bestseller; I had Wednesdays with Frannie, my mother's name being Frances.

After lunch, we'd sit on the back porch overlooking a horse pasture and watch the clouds, nebulous puffs of angelic DNA that always spurred conversation. Like two old friends who had journeyed down the road of life together, we'd talk candidly about what was on our minds. Nothing and nobody was off the table. Inevitably, the conversation drifted to living and dying. My mother had made her peace with God, but questions remained. Now after the hike, I had some perspective if not answers for her.

"I don't know why God keeps me alive. I lived my life. I'm ready for the next step," my mother would always opine with a puzzled look. My answer was always the same.

"One thing I learned on the trail is that we're here for a purpose, even if we don't know what it is. Just like Pop was in the nursing home, you're here for a specific purpose. It may be a friend, a family member, or a stranger, but it's all connected just as we're all connected to God. All part of the great mystery."

"You mean the divine plan," she would joke, rolling her eyes.

"What do you think it's like in heaven?" she would ask wistfully as a follow-up question.

"A place of unparalleled beauty and unbounded love where dreams come true. A place that humans have a hard time imagining. You see what God does with nature. Imagine what he can do with dreams," I would espouse philosophically.

"Sounds like something from the '60s and your hippie friends," she would laugh before gleefully rehashing my college years from her perspective. Growing up in a deeply religious Polish family, my mother had difficulty embracing concepts outside the Catholic faith, or in other words thinking outside the spiritual box. However, over time, my trail mantras about connectedness and coincidence (synchronicity) were making headway. She was gradually beginning to see the universe in a different light.

My mother's skepticism about my new spiritual identity was blunted by the sudden arrival of my father's WWII footlocker. For nearly seventy years, the small trunk had been missing in action. My father last saw it in September 1944 before boarding a troop transport for Peleliu.

Over the Memorial Day weekend in 2013, I

received a phone call from a gentleman who lived about two hours away, asking me if I was related to H. J. Travers, who had been in the service. He had an old footlocker with my father's name, service number, and the word EPIC (code name for New Caledonia, the staging area for the Pacific island campaign) stenciled on the top and sides. He had purchased the footlocker over twenty years ago at an antique shop and was going to sell it at a yard sale. Thinking it might have sentimental value to a family member, he tracked me down through my father's obituary and the Internet. That evening I raced to his house with a goodwill offering to rescue the heirloom.

"Just the universe reaching out with a friendly wink," I said to my mother after giving her the footlocker. With tears in her eyes, she ran her hands over the top, gently rubbing my father's name, and peered inside.

"You can have it. It's your inheritance. I have no place to put it," my mother sniffled after a few minutes. Later on, she admitted to me the footlocker held too many bittersweet memories.

During my last visit before her death, we sat outside in the garden of the assisted living facility, now her home due to her failing health. My mother was unusually quiet. Surrounded by nature, an inner peace had settled over her countenance as if she knew her time was at hand. In her lap, she had a plastic bag containing photos of her parents and siblings, most dating to the early 1940s. One by one, she extracted the images with a convivial monologue. When she handed me a picture of Sister Regina in her religious habit, I gasped silently. My hand trembled. The facial features of the twenty-year-old nun strikingly resembled the girl from Laurel Fork Creek.

With a final picture of my father, my mother relived their good times while stoically staring off into the distance of an adjacent cornfield.

"You've been truly blessed. Despite the tragedy of Alzheimer's, you have triumphed," I intoned reverently, tenderly holding her hand.

"How so?" she replied meekly.

"Because of your ordeal, you have known divine love. You have peeked behind the curtain and glimpsed the face of God." My mother gently squeezed my hand in silence and sighed. For once in her life, she knew that I had been right.

Until her death, my mother prayed daily, updating her prayer list with new names and adding two requests of her own. She wanted to die in her sleep and didn't want to die alone. I always reassured her that no one dies alone, reciting my encounters with my guardian angels. As for the "sleep" part, she was on her own.

"God's busy with a trillion prayers an hour. Be more specific. Give him some times and dates," I'd joke before retelling my tale about Circuit Rider and his advice. She was listening.

On July 24, a week after our last talk, my mother crossed over in her sleep. At the time, she had been listening to the weekly musical worship service. Surrounded by her new friends, she gently closed her eyes for the last time. Her prayer had been answered.

As with my father, I was the first family member to arrive. I was immediately ushered to my mother's bedroom where her body had been taken. I sat by her side while the minister from the worship service prayed quietly in the background. There was a divine stillness in the air that reminded me of my mystical nights on the trail. For a brief second, angels with perfumed wings filled the air. I could hear the rustle and smell the flowers. My mother was finally standing on that sacred mountain and reaching out to touch the heavens.

Gently clenching her warm hand, I recalled our last month together and remembered that today was Wednesday, our day together. While hundreds of memories flooded my mind, I smiled when I recalled our last talk. After telling her my dream about Pop and the blue headband, she surprised me with her own story. In one of her recent dreams, she saw my father and me hiking in a forest. I was about ten years old wearing my Davey Crockett hat, and my dad was a young soldier dressed in his army khakis. After she finished, we simply looked at each other with tight smiles and nodded before returning to study the clouds. I didn't ask about any blue headbands.

Climbing the steps to the pulpit once again for the eulogy, I gazed at the familiar faces from my father's funeral. Although there was no military flavor to the service, the Stars and Stripes should have been draped over my mother's casket. During the war, she had worked as a "Rosie the Riveter" and nurtured a wounded war veteran back to health as a young bride. That was worthy of a medal or two for an unsung patriot. Fulfilling my mother's wish, my youngest daughter sang another emotional rendition of "Ave Maria." Tears filled my eyes knowing that my mother heard every word.

My mother was buried next to my father. They were finally resting side by side as they wanted. As I walked away from the gravesite with Brite and my daughters, I was filled with an overwhelming calmness. My mother's physical and emotional suffering had been painful to watch. Yet, I took comfort in knowing that she had weathered the "darkest night of the soul" and emerged with a stronger faith in God. I knew that she had found the heaven of her dreams.

Any tinge of sadness that I felt was for myself. I was going to sorely miss Wednesday afternoons. I only wished that I had those conversations with my father. That evening I once again went outside and watched the stars in the summer sky. They appeared to be twinkling brighter than ever. This time I didn't need a celestial event to reveal the divine truth. In my heart and soul, I knew that nature was not the handiwork of God but the hand of God. During my hike, God and I held hands many times. With my mother's passing, I also realized that my spiritual journey had come full circle. I had lived my father's dream and followed my mother's advice. "Go outside and play," I heard her voice echo across the heavens that night. I was glad that I did.

Epilogue
Beyond Katahdin

Pursue some path, however narrow and crooked, in which you can walk in love and reverence. —Henry David Thoreau

We are stardust. We are golden. And we've got to get ourselves back to the garden. —Joni Mitchell from the song *"Woodstock."*

Transcendent moments on the mountains transformed my life. Nature became my religion, the mountains—my cathedral, the valleys—my pew, the trees—my congregation, the rivers—my baptismal font, and the Appalachian Trail—my spiritual home. I took the road less traveled, the essence of every pilgrimage, and found a new spiritual identity. After summiting Katahdin, my spiritual Everest, the challenge now was to keep moving forward spiritually. And the only way to do that was to keep hiking. Brite and I hiked the Adirondacks and the Grand Canyon among others. I frequented hiking trails near my house. With the AT just two hours from my house, I enjoyed day hikes and the occasional overnight backpacking trip. It was fulfilling, but I needed more spiritual voltage to recharge my spiritual battery. I wanted and needed to mountain dance beyond Katahdin.

I was ready to hit the trail for an extended

stay, but the trail was elusive. I quickly discovered that senior hikers are in short supply and shorter demand. Not wanting to hike alone, I scoured hiking websites for partners. Fortunately, the Nashville Backpackers, led by the original Rain Man, who was completing his AT section-hike, came to my rescue. For five summers, I hiked various sections of the AT for a week or two at a time. There was no more convivial and congenial group ever to hike the AT. During one of those trail communions, the chance to break bread with new trail friends, this book was conceived.

Following completion of Herm's Hike, people urged me to write a book about my transcendent experience. I dismissed the idea outright. There were already enough AT books, mostly compilations of trail journals and diaries, to stock a library. Besides, I didn't want to merely publish an AT journal, I wanted to write an AT story. *But what could I offer my readers?*

When a fellow hiker suggested that my journey could give hope and comfort to families struggling with personal tragedy, I decided to write. If I reached only one person, it would be worth the effort. While my story was intertwined with a number of stories on and off the trail, the literary trailheads were easy to find. The love story of my parents was the starting point. The love story of two childhood friends, who eventually married and confronted Alzheimer's in their late fifties, was the inspiration for finishing. At times, the writing was as emotionally challenging as hiking the AT. Like hiking one step at a time, I took it one word at a time. In many sentences, it proved to be one teardrop at a time.

Alzheimer's and other diseases that slowly rob the

mind like a thief in the night are some of the most hideous plagues to confront mankind. Writers of the macabre, such as Edgar Allan Poe and Stephen King, could not have invented or imagined a more evil fate where condemned souls are trapped in a frightening fog of forgetfulness and loneliness to scream in silent anguish. Our memories are our human footprints, our landmarks on our earthly journey. They are the essence of our spirit. Without them, we are wisps of clouds, nothing more than mortal ghosts. For those who have forgotten themselves, it's our moral duty to remember their lives as sacred points of light.

When a disease empties the mind and leaves a crumbing physical shell, there still exists a sacred tabernacle that houses the divine light, a cosmic dot reflecting the majesty and mystery of God. By embracing the mystery of human suffering, we fulfill our spiritual destiny by manifesting our inherent divine love through compassion. When that happens, we don't become God. We become God's lover.

As for myself, my accumulated good karma resulted in an unconditional absolution from the baseball gods. In 2011, I finally made it to the Big Leagues as a ballpark tour guide for the Baltimore Orioles. Adhering to my spiritual regime, I still gaze at the stars and chase the clouds, quite certain there are a few more celestial dots to connect before my cosmic portrait is finished. Herm's Hike and this book were merely two more dots. I continue to hike along my spiritual path, guided by points of white light instead of white blazes. To my fellow travelers, my advice is simple: As you journey down the road of life, hike with your angels and hike in peace. Namaste!

About the Author

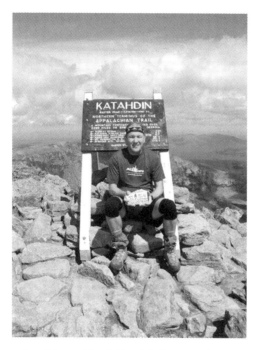

Atop Mount Katahdin with the sacred stone.

Paul J. Travers received a BA from the University of Maryland in English and an MA from Pepperdine University in Human Resources Management. Following graduation, he served as an amphibious armor officer in the US Marine Corps. A former park ranger and historian with the Maryland Park Service, he is also the author of *Eyewitness to Infamy (An Oral History of Pearl Harbor)*, *The Patapsco: Baltimore's River of History*, *The Flight of the Shadow Drummer*, and *The Cowgirl and the Colts*.

Over the past decade, he has been involved with

various historical and environmental groups. Proving that "60" is the new "16," he has fulfilled his childhood dream of becoming a drummer in a rock n' roll band. After sixty seasons, he finally reached the Big Leagues as a ballpark tour guide with the Baltimore Orioles. He continues to hike the Appalachian Trail.

If you liked this book, you might also like:

Application of Impossible Things
by Natalie Sudman
A Quest of Transcendence
by Jolene and Jason Tierney
Divine Gifts of Healing
by Cat Baldwin
Embracing Your Human Journey
by Janie Wells
Finding your way in the Spiritual Age
by Dan Bird
Heaven Here on Earth
by Curt Melliger
Headless Chicken
by Manuela Stoerzer

For more information about any of the above titles, soon to be released titles,
or other items in our catalog, write, phone or visit our website:
Ozark Mountain Publishing, LLC
PO Box 754, Huntsville, AR 72740
479-738-2348
www.ozarkmt.com

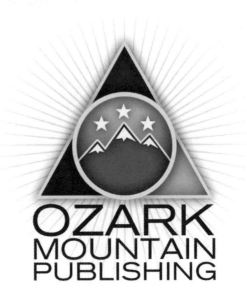

OZARK
MOUNTAIN
PUBLISHING

For more information about any of the titles published by Ozark Mountain Publishing, Inc., soon to be released titles, or other items in our catalog, write, phone or visit our website:

Ozark Mountain Publishing, Inc.

PO Box 754

Huntsville, AR 72740

479-738-2348/800-935-0045

www.ozarkmt.com

Other Books by Ozark Mountain Publishing, Inc.

Dolores Cannon
A Soul Remembers Hiroshima
Between Death and Life
Conversations with Nostradamus,
    Volume I, II, III
The Convoluted Universe -Book One,
    Two, Three, Four, Five
The Custodians
Five Lives Remembered
Jesus and the Essenes
Keepers of the Garden
Legacy from the Stars
The Legend of Starcrash
The Search for Hidden Sacred Knowledge
They Walked with Jesus
The Three Waves of Volunteers and the
    New Earth
Aron Abrahamsen
Holiday in Heaven
Out of the Archives – Earth Changes
James Ream Adams
Little Steps
Justine Alessi & M. E. McMillan
Rebirth of the Oracle
Kathryn/Patrick Andries
Naked in Public
Kathryn Andries
The Big Desire
Dream Doctor
Soul Choices: Six Paths to Find Your Life
    Purpose
Soul Choices: Six Paths to Fulfilling
    Relationships
Patrick Andries
Owners Manual for the Mind
Cat Baldwin
Divine Gifts of Healing
Dan Bird
Finding Your Way in the Spiritual Age
Waking Up in the Spiritual Age
Julia Cannon
Soul Speak – The Language of Your Body
Ronald Chapman
Seeing True
Albert Cheung
The Emperor's Stargate
Jack Churchward
Lifting the Veil on the Lost Continent of
    Mu
The Stone Tablets of Mu
Sherri Cortland

Guide Group Fridays
Raising Our Vibrations for the New Age
Spiritual Tool Box
Windows of Opportunity
Patrick De Haan
The Alien Handbook
Paulinne Delcour-Min
Spiritual Gold
Holly Ice
Divine Fire
Joanne DiMaggio
Edgar Cayce and the Unfulfilled Destiny
    of Thomas Jefferson Reborn
Anthony DeNino
The Power of Giving and Gratitude
Michael Dennis
Morning Coffee with God
God's Many Mansions
Carolyn Greer Daly
Opening to Fullness of Spirit
Anita Holmes
Twidders
Aaron Hoopes
Reconnecting to the Earth
Victoria Hunt
Kiss the Wind
Patricia Irvine
In Light and In Shade
Kevin Killen
Ghosts and Me
Diane Lewis
From Psychic to Soul
Donna Lynn
From Fear to Love
Maureen McGill
Baby It's You
Maureen McGill & Nola Davis
Live from the Other Side
Curt Melliger
Heaven Here on Earth
Henry Michaelson
And Jesus Said – A Conversation
Dennis Milner
Kosmos
Andy Myers
Not Your Average Angel Book
Guy Needler
Avoiding Karma
Beyond the Source – Book 1, Book 2
The Anne Dialogues

For more information about any of the above titles, soon to be released titles,
or other items in our catalog, write, phone or visit our website:
PO Box 754, Huntsville, AR 72740
479-738-2348/800-935-0045
www.ozarkmt.com

Other Books by Ozark Mountain Publishing, Inc.

The Curators
The History of God
The Origin Speaks
James Nussbaumer
And Then I Knew My Abundance
The Master of Everything
Mastering Your Own Spiritual Freedom
Living Your Dram, Not Someone Else's
Sherry O'Brian
Peaks and Valleys
Riet Okken
The Liberating Power of Emotions
Gabrielle Orr
Akashic Records: One True Love
Let Miracles Happen
Victor Parachin
Sit a Bit
Nikki Pattillo
A Spiritual Evolution
Children of the Stars
Rev. Grant H. Pealer
A Funny Thing Happened on the
    Way to Heaven
Worlds Beyond Death
Victoria Pendragon
Born Healers
Feng Shui from the Inside, Out
Sleep Magic
The Sleeping Phoenix
Being In A Body
Michael Perlin
Fantastic Adventures in Metaphysics
Walter Pullen
Evolution of the Spirit
Debra Rayburn
Let's Get Natural with Herbs
Charmian Redwood
A New Earth Rising
Coming Home to Lemuria
David Rivinus
Always Dreaming
Richard Rowe
Imagining the Unimaginable
Exploring the Divine Library
M. Don Schorn
Elder Gods of Antiquity
Legacy of the Elder Gods
Gardens of the Elder Gods
Reincarnation...Stepping Stones of Life
Garnet Schulhauser
Dance of Eternal Rapture

Dance of Heavenly Bliss
Dancing Forever with Spirit
Dancing on a Stamp
Manuella Stoerzer
Headless Chicken
Annie Stillwater Gray
Education of a Guardian Angel
The Dawn Book
Work of a Guardian Angel
Joys of a Guardian Angel
Blair Styra
Don't Change the Channel
Who Catharted
Natalie Sudman
Application of Impossible Things
L.R. Sumpter
Judy's Story
The Old is New
We Are the Creators
Artur Tradevosyan
Croton
Jim Thomas
Tales from the Trance
Jolene and Jason Tierney
A Quest of Transcendence
Paul Travers
Dancing with the Mountains
Nicholas Vesey
Living the Life-Force
Janie Wells
Embracing the Human Journey
Payment for Passage
Dennis Wheatley/ Maria Wheatley
The Essential Dowsing Guide
Maria Wheatley
Druidic Soul Star Astrology
Jacquelyn Wiersma
The Zodiac Recipe
Sherry Wilde
The Forgotten Promise
Lyn Willmott
A Small Book of Comfort
Beyond all Boundaries Book 1
Stuart Wilson & Joanna Prentis
Atlantis and the New Consciousness
Beyond Limitations
The Essenes -Children of the Light
The Magdalene Version
Power of the Magdalene
Robert Winterhalter
The Healing Christ

For more information about any of the above titles, soon to be released titles,
or other items in our catalog, write, phone or visit our website:
PO Box 754, Huntsville, AR 72740
479-738-2348/800-935-0045
www.ozarkmt.com